Myocardial Imaging

Peter R. McLaughlin, M.D.
Associate Director, Cardiovascular Unit
Co-Director, Nuclear Cardiology Laboratory
Toronto General Hospital
Associate Professor, University of Toronto

John E. Morch, M.D.
Department of Nuclear Medicine
Royal Jubilee Hospital
Victoria, British Columbia

Manuscript prepared with the editorial assistance of
Medi-Edit Limited, Toronto

ADDISON-WESLEY PUBLISHING COMPANY, INC.
Medical/Nursing Division, Menlo Park, California
Reading, Massachusetts • Don Mills, Ontario • Wokingham, U.K.
Amsterdam • Sydney • Singapore • Tokyo • Mexico City
Bogota • Santiago • San Juan

Sponsoring Editor: Katherine Pitcoff
Production Coordinator: Greg Hubit

Library of Congress Cataloging in Publication Data

Main entry under title:

Myocardial imaging.

  Bibliography: p.
  Includes index.
  1. Radioisotope scanning.   2. Heart—Diseases—
Diagnosis.   3. Angiocardiography.   I. McLaughlin,
Peter R.   II. Morch, John E.
RC683.5.R33M933   1985   616.1'207575   84-21720
ISBN 0-201-14177-9

ISBN 0-201-14177-9

ABCDEFGHIJ-MA-898765

The authors and publishers have exerted every effort to ensure that drug selection and dosage formulations and composition of formulas set forth in this text are in accord with current recommendations and practice at the time of publication. However, in view of ongoing research, changes in government regulations, the reformulation of nutritional products, and the constant flow of information relating to drug therapy and drug reactions, the reader is urged to check product information on composition or the package insert for each drug for any change in indications of dosage and for added warnings and precautions. This is particularly important where the recommended agent is a new and/or infrequently employed drug.

Addison-Wesley Publishing Company, Inc.
Medical/Nursing Division
2725 Sand Hill Road
Menlo Park, California 94025

To Rhys McLaughlin and Sandy Morch

Contributors

Stephen L. Bacharach, Ph.D.
Division of Nuclear Medicine
Clinical Center
National Institutes of Health
Bethesda, Maryland

Frederick J. Bonte, M.D.
Professor of Radiology and Dean
Southwestern Medical School
The University of Texas Health Science
    Center at Dallas, Texas

Jeffrey S. Borer, M.D.
Cardiology Division
Department of Medicine
New York Hospital–Cornell Medical Center
New York, New York

L. Maximilian Buja, M.D.
Professor of Pathology
Southwestern Medical School
The University of Texas Health Science
    Center at Dallas, Texas

Graham J. Davies, M.B.
Royal Postgraduate Medical School
University of London
Cardiovascular Research Unit
Hammersmith Hospital
London, England

Maurice N. Druck, M.D.
Staff Cardiologist
Director of Non-Invasive Cardiology
    and Nuclear Cardiology Laboratory
Toronto Western Hospital
Toronto, Ontario, Canada

David H. Feiglin, M.B.B.S., B.Sc.,
    FRCP(C), MACS
Division of Nuclear Medicine
The Cleveland Clinic Foundation
Cleveland, Ohio

Gary F. Gates, M.D.
Clinical Associate Professor of Diagnostic
    Radiology
University of Oregon School of Medicine
Director of Nuclear Medicine
Good Samaritan Hospital and
    Medical Center
Portland, Oregon

Michael V. Green, M.S.
Division of Nuclear Medicine
Clinical Center
National Institutes of Health
Bethesda, Maryland

Victor F. Huckell, M.D.
Assistant Professor of Medicine
University of British Columbia
Vancouver, British Columbia, Canada

William J. Kostuk, M.D.
Cardiac Investigation Unit
University Hospital
London, Ontario, Canada

Samuel E. Lewis, M.D.
Assistant Professor of Pathology
Southwestern Medical School
The University of Texas Health Science
    Center at Dallas, Texas

Peter R. McLaughlin, M.D.
Associate Director, Cardiovascular
    Unit, and Co-Director
Nuclear Cardiology Laboratory
Toronto General Hospital
Associate Professor
University of Toronto
Toronto, Ontario, Canada

Attilio Maseri, M.D.
Royal Postgraduate Medical School
University of London
London, England

John E. Morch, M.D.
Department of Nuclear Medicine
Royal Jubilee Hospital
Victoria, British Columbia, Canada

Robert W. Parkey, M.D.
Professor and Chairman
Department of Radiology
Southwestern Medical School
The University of Texas Health Science
    Center at Dallas, Texas

Oberdan Parodi, M.D.
CNR Institute of Clinical Physiology
University of Pisa
Pisa, Italy

Frans J. Wackers, M.D.
Associate Professor of Diagnostic Radiology
    and Medicine
Yale University School of Medicine
New Haven, Connecticut

James T. Willerson, M.D.
Professor of Medicine
Director, Cardiology Division
Department of Internal Medicine
The University of Texas Health Science
    Center at Dallas, Texas

Preface

Nuclear cardiology has developed rapidly over the past decade and is now a firmly established discipline within cardiology and nuclear medicine. These developments have been accompanied by new technologies, a new group of subspecialists who devote their professional time to this area, and new concepts and language that are not immediately familiar to the practicing physician and student alike. The techniques and pharmaceuticals used for imaging the myocardium are several, and the hardware and computer software used to analyze studies are undergoing constant change and upgrading.

The aim of this book has been to present this diverse field in a manner that will make it useful for the clinician. Contributors include several of the best-known figures in the field, who have made significant contributions to the development of nuclear cardiology. They have summarized their particular areas of expertise with the objective of providing the reader with a review of the indications, limitations, and clinical relevance of each imaging technique. In rapidly changing areas, future directions are indicated, but emphasis has been placed on what has been shown to be clinically useful and practical. The many illustrations provide the clinician with examples of some of the more important applications of imaging. Obviously, certain applications, such as radionuclide angiography, cannot be adequately illustrated in a printed text.

The book has been kept short enough to be useful for the physician or surgeon who does not want a great amount of technical detail, but rather a concise presentation of the uses and limitations of these techniques. For those not directly involved in nuclear cardiology, this will assist in the selection of patients who can benefit from these studies, and contribute to a better integration of results in the decision-making process.

Peter R. McLaughlin, M.D.
John E. Morch, M.D.
Editors

Contents

Introduction

More than half a century has passed since Blumgart and Weiss (1927) first followed the passage of a radiotracer through the heart. Almost thirty years later, Burch and coworkers (1955) began to use rubidium-86 to image myocardial infarction. In the early sixties, Carr and associates (1962) demonstrated the localization of mercury labeled compounds in acute infarction, and Evans, Gunton, et al. (1965) introduced myocardial imaging with radiolabeled fatty acids. The use of exercise as a physiologic stress, first described by Zaret, Strauss, et al. (1973), was a most important advance that has greatly influenced the clinical utility of myocardial perfusion imaging. Of equal importance was the introduction of ECG-gated equilibrium blood pool cardiac imaging (Zaret, Strauss, et al., 1971) for the assessment of ventricular function, and its evolution to exercise radionuclide angiography (Borer, Bacharach, et al., 1977).

The rapid emergence of nuclear cardiology as a distinct clinical field has been made possible by three basic developments. First, introduction of the gamma camera by Anger in the early 1960s allowed the rapid acquisition of scintillation events, with both spatial and temporal resolution. More recent improvements in resolution and the mobility of cameras have permitted the acquisition of high-quality images at the bedside of critically ill patients. Second, the introduction of clinically safe radiopharmaceuticals and labeling techniques has permitted exploration by different avenues of cardiac function and physiology. For example, technetium-99m pyrophosphate can be used to identify acute myocardial infarction, thallium-201 to assess relative myocardial perfusion at rest and during exercise, and technetium-99m labeled red blood cells to study ventricular function. Third, the introduction of small dedicated computers linked to the gamma camera has permitted rapid data collection in digitized format that allows for more sophisticated and quantitative data analysis. The rapidity with which new computer programs have been developed over the past six years is breathtaking for the noncomputer-oriented clinician, who cannot help but wonder whether he or she can "keep up" in this area.

The purpose of this book is to simplify myocardial imaging for the clinician and to present an up-to-date review of current knowledge in a manner that will make it useful in day-to-day practice. To accomplish this goal, the text has been divided into a "basic" first chapter, in which principles of radionuclide techniques and equipment are described, followed by clinical chapters in which imaging for the different disease entities is considered. This arrangement departs from the usual presentation of this field by technique alone. It organizes essential information in a more clinically relevant format—patients presenting with their particular disease entity.

Before consideration is given to imaging by specific disease states, it is helpful to define the different techniques:

1. *"Hot spot" imaging of acute infarction.* Technetium-99m pyrophosphate labels acutely infarcted myocardium as a "hot spot."

2. *"Cold spot" imaging.* Thallium-201 labels areas of infarction, ischemia, and fibrosis as "cold spots."

3. *Radionuclide angiography.* Technetium-99m labeled red blood cells are used for "gated" radionuclide angiography, or followed as a bolus through the heart for first pass radionuclide imaging. Both provide angiograms for assessment of ventricular wall motion and ventricular ejection fractions.

4. *Coronary flow (investigational).* Xenon-133 or labeled microspheres are injected directly into the coronary arteries at the time of cardiac catheterization, for measurement of coronary perfusion.

5. *Labeled platelets, leukocytes, and fatty acids (investigational).* This technique may prove useful for specific conditions, such as infective endocarditis or graft thrombosis, and for the assessment of myocardial metabolism.

6. *Positron imaging (investigational).* This imaging technique has a promising future as a research tool. It requires a special camera and production facilities, permitting short half-life imaging and labeling of specific metabolic substrates.

The first three techniques are currently being used clinically and are generally available, and we will concentrate on their use in a variety of cardiovascular conditions. The last three investigational techniques will be discussed only briefly.

References

Blumgart, H. L.; and Weiss, S. 1927. Studies on the velocity of blood flow: VII. The pulmonary circulation time in normal resting individuals. *J. Clin. Invest.* 4:399–407.

Borer, J. S.; Bacharach, S. L.; Green, M. V., et al. 1977. Real-time radionuclide cineangiography in the noninvasive evaluation of global and regional left ventricular function at rest and during exercise in patients with coronary artery disease. *N. Engl. J. Med.* 296:839–44.

Burch, G. E.; Threefoot, S. A.; and Ray, C. T. 1955. The rate of disappearance of Rb[86] from the plasma, the biological decay rates of Rb[86], and the applicability of Rb[86] as a tracer of potassium in man with and without chronic congestive failure. *J. Lab. Clin. Med.* 45:371–78.

Carr, E. A.; Beierwaltes, W. H.; Patno, M. E., et al. 1962. The detection of experimental myocardial infarcts by photoscanning. *Am. Heart J.* 64:650–60.

Evans, J. R.; Gunton, R. W.; Baker, R. G., et al. 1965. Use of radioiodinated fatty acid for photoscans of the heart. *Circ. Res.* 16:1–10.

Zaret, B. L.; Strauss, H. W.; Hurley, P. J., et al. 1971. A non-invasive scintiphotographic method for detecting regional ventricular dysfunction in man. *N. Engl. J. Med.* 284:1165–70.

Zaret, B. L.; Strauss, H. W.; Martin, N. D., et al. 1973. Non-invasive regional myocardial perfusion with radioactive potassium: Study of patients at rest, with exercise and during angina pectoris. *N. Engl. J. Med.* 288:809–12.

1 Isotopes, Instrumentation, and Techniques

David H. Feiglin, M.B.B.S., B.Sc., FRCP(C), MACS

Division of Nuclear Medicine
The Cleveland Clinic Foundation
Cleveland, Ohio

The author expresses his thanks to Dr. E. W. Spiers for technical assistance.

Clinical imaging of the myocardium involves, primarily, perfusion or thallium scanning (Strauss and Pitt, 1977), functional or gated nuclear angiography, and infarct avid or "hot spot" scanning (McLaughlin, Coates, et al., 1975). In the performance of these studies, consideration must be given to instrumentation, the computer, radiopharmaceuticals, techniques, and image processing and display. This chapter will concentrate on these areas and provide explanations of relevant concepts.

INSTRUMENTATION

Instrumentation for cardiac imaging involves the use of either a gamma camera or a scintillation probe unit. The scintillation probe unit (Groch, Gottlieb, et al., 1976), or "nuclear stethoscope," while allowing a significantly higher sensitivity than the gamma camera for a given dose of radiopharmaceutical, does not provide images. In practical terms, it is inappropriate as a first piece of imaging equipment. The scintillation probe unit is a rather specialized or dedicated unit best reserved for areas in which other imaging equipment (gamma camera) is also available. It has as its major advantage the capability to provide some evaluation of cardiac function, such as ejection fraction, with doses of radioactivity less than those required for the gamma camera (Ashburn, Schelbert, et al., 1978) at a lower initial cost. This discussion, however, will focus on the more commonly used gamma camera.

The Gamma Camera

Commercial gamma cameras consist of a sodium iodide radiation detector coupled with light pipes to an array of photomultiplier tubes. Gamma ray interaction in the sodium iodide crystal produces light scintillations that are detected by the photomultiplier tubes and converted to electrical signals. The sum of the outputs from all photomultiplier tubes provides a Z signal proportional to the energy of the gamma rays which can be used to reject the scattered gamma rays of decreased energy. The scattering of gamma rays is a result of their physical interaction with matter (in this case, the body) and consequent loss of energy and change in direction of travel. If the scattered gamma rays were counted, the imaging equipment would assume their source of origin to be from the point of interaction and not from their actual source. This misinformation can lead to significant image degradation.

The individual photomultiplier signals are fed to a "position computer." Photomultipliers close to the scintillation source have larger outputs than those remote from it, and this generates X and Y positional signals (Figure 1-1).

Different signal processing techniques are available in commercial cameras, such as resistor matrix and delay lines (not currently used). Theoretically, delay line technology offers improved resolution, while resistor matrix provides higher counting efficiency. Currently available

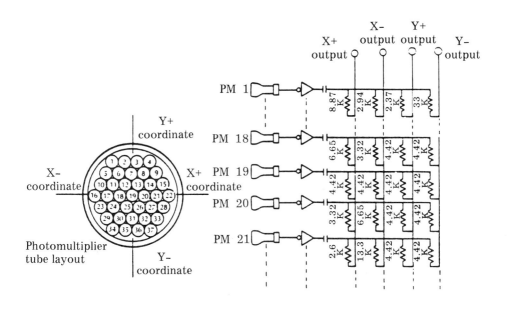

Figure 1-1 A detector resistor matrix that demonstrates how the amplified signals from the photomultiplier tubes are applied to a resistor matrix that, in turn, combines them into four positioning signals, X^+, X^-, Y^+, Y^-, which are proportional to the weighted sums of the inputs.

"state of the art" cameras use the resistor matrix system with an analog signal output. (Some recent commercial cameras can provide a direct digital output that is fed into a computer; the computer is an integral part of the system. This capability circumvents the problems of analog signals and gives improved performance.) For nuclear angiograms, fast counting rates and, to a lesser extent, resolving capability are of primary interest. With thallium imaging, the count rates are less critical, so optimization of resolution is more desirable.

The trend in commercial equipment is toward the matrix processing technology. With this type of equipment, rates of 20,000 to 30,000 counts per second (cps) can be achieved without significant data loss. With rates up to 150,000 cps, measurable but usually acceptable data losses occur. The count losses may be significant only in the range of very high rates, in excess of 100,000 cps. Computing techniques that attempt to correct for this problem are available. However, where high count rates are needed, such as in first pass studies, a multicrystal camera can be used to overcome the problem—although at the expense of resolution loss and at an equipment cost higher than that for the single crystal camera. For practical purposes, a standard processing gamma camera remains quite appropriate for most nuclear cardiac studies.

The trend in camera design has been toward an ever-increasing size in the field of view or area that the camera can image at any one time. Early models that are still available and some mobile cameras have a 25 cm field of view. Sizes have increased to 35–40 cm, and some newer cameras offer a field of view 50 cm or greater. The number of photomultiplier tubes varies from 37 in the smaller cameras to 61, 75, and even 91, the increasing numbers providing improved intrinsic resolution. With the larger number of tubes, problems in stability, uniformity, and servicing can arise. When a collimator is added, however, the improvement in resolution may not be clinically significant and may not justify the added cost of, say, upgrading from a 37- to a 75-tube system. Cameras are also available as either fixed or mobile systems. The latter usually have a small field of view (25 cm), although some of the newer mobile camera systems provide a larger head.

These systems have advantages and disadvantages. From a cardiological viewpoint, all radionuclides of practical use are of low energy, that is, less than 160 kev, and the organ of interest is less than 25 cm in diameter. A small field of view camera without high energy requirements is therefore adequate.

The clinician must decide whether a mobile or a stationary system is more appropriate for his or her purpose. At present there is only marginal improvement in the stability and performance of stationary systems as opposed to mobile units. In summary, the choice of a camera for cardiac imaging would weigh toward a mobile camera because of its portability.

Like many imaging modalities, gamma cameras have limitations that are discussed by experts in technical terms. Five of these terms will be reviewed to assist the reader's understanding: uniformity, spatial resolution, linearity, energy resolution, and count rate capability (National Electrical Manufacturers Association, 1980).

Uniformity Uniformity relates to the camera's ability to provide a uniform response to a uniform output. Unfortunately, total uniformity is not yet a practical reality; all cameras "color" or modify their output to some degree. For example, if (1) a uniform source of radioactivity (2–5 mCi) is placed adjacent to a collimated camera head, or if (2) a point source of activity (approximately 100 uCi) is set at some distance (150–200 cm) from an uncollimated head, the camera will show a varying count response in varying positions. In the first case the system response will be evaluated clinically, and in the second the photomultiplier tube/crystal response without collimator will be tested. Nonuniformity can be minimized by careful tuning of the camera. A variance of ±5% across 80% of the field of view is not unusual. To maintain this uniformity, the tubes around the edge may have to be tuned differently, which usually gives rise to an "edge packing" effect with a significant lack of uniformity. In all scanning procedures, the organ(s) of interest should be visualized away from the edge of the field of view.

To maintain other operating parameters, some cameras forego the initial uniformity response and rely on on-board microprocessors to provide appropriate corrections. Other techniques involve computer correction of data after collection. Whatever technique is used, one must be careful to ensure that data are not erroneously introduced or deleted. With the processing currently available, almost perfect uniformity can be obtained, but in some systems processing can lead to erroneous addition or deletion of data.

There is no substitute for careful and regular tuning of the gamma camera. Flood correction techniques alone should not be relied upon for this purpose; instead, these should be performed in conjunction with tuning whenever necessary (Figure 1-2).

Spatial Resolution Spatial resolution is a measure of a camera's ability to discriminate between two point sources of activity. Most camera tests are performed using ^{57}Co, which has a gamma emission energy of 120 kev. Currently available cameras without a collimator can intrinsically resolve 2 mm lead bars in a phantom under test conditions. However, resolution

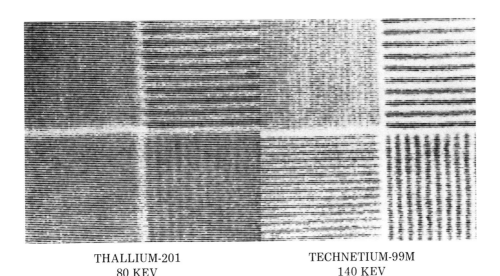

THALLIUM-201   TECHNETIUM-99M
80 KEV   140 KEV

Figure 1-2 Camera resolution at 80 and 140 kev. Reading clockwise from the upper right-hand corner, lead bars are at 4.8 mm, 4.0 mm, 3.2 mm, and 2.4 mm. It is possible to see all the bars on the technetium image, whereas the thallium image resolves only the 4.8 and 4.0 mm bars. This response is normal for all Anger cameras and indicates that the camera resolving capability is better with 140 kev (viz. 2.4 mm) than with 80 kev (viz. 4.0 mm). Images are taken from a 256 × 256 flood collection.

capability is in turn affected by collimator parameters which lead to a net effective equipment resolution of about 4 to 5 mm at the collimator face. Spatial resolution is a function of the organ-to-collimator face distance, energy of the radionuclide used, and type of collimator. Performance comparisons for imaging equipment can be accurately made only when identical test procedures are used. In practice, these data are not always easily obtained. Resolution specifications, such as those obtained using ^{57}Co (120 kev), are generally close to those obtained with ^{99m}Tc, but are vastly different from those for lower-energy ^{201}Tl (80 kev) or higher-energy ^{131}I (364 kev). What may be visualized on a clinical image obtained with technetium might well not be seen with thallium, since camera systems currently in use perform optimally in the 120–150 kev range (Figure 1-3).

Linearity Linearity of a camera system concerns its ability to output a straight line or edge in response to a corresponding input. Some variance always exists, but a system should not be used if, after appropriate data collection using a phantom, linearity cannot be demonstrated. A nonlinear

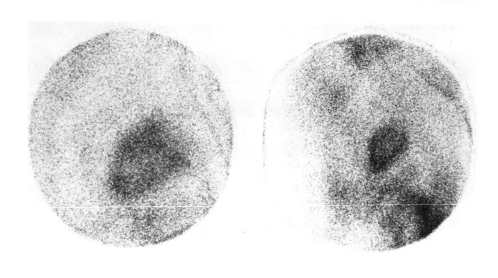

Figure 1-3 Rest 45° left anterior oblique thallium images in the same patient. The left-hand image was performed with a high-resolution converging collimator and the right-hand image with a high-resolution parallel-hole collimator on a GCA 402 Toshiba large field of view camera. Both images contain 400K counts, the left image taking 50% of the collection time of the right. Note the geometric distortion of the left image compared to the right. The data from the right image can be easily magnified either at the camera source or by the ADCs during input or during data analysis.

response will lead to significant geometric distortion of images. Careful tuning of the camera system can optimize linearity, and some new camera systems actually perform on-line linearity corrections.

Energy Resolution The ability of a scintillation device to discern different gamma energies relates to energy resolution. Figures in the range of 10% to 12% are considered acceptable. Higher figures indicate deterioration or less than optimal systems, with reduced ability to discriminate scattered radiation from nonscattered radiation, resulting in an image of poorer quality.

The tuning of a camera is usually a compromise among optimal resolution, uniformity, and linearity; it is impossible to optimize all parameters. Many nuclear physicians prefer to optimize uniformity to provide the best clinical images.

Count Rate Capability The ideal gamma camera should maintain performance characteristics independent of count rate input. No detectable difference in image quality should be discernible between scans collected at 1,000 cps and those collected at 100,000 cps. A finite period of time is required by camera electronics to process each signal as it occurs. During this "dead time," which varies from 1–2 up to 10 microseconds depending on the camera, the camera is unavailable for processing another signal.

At high counting rates, therefore, the camera cannot detect a significant fraction of the incoming gamma rays, and thus may distort the images because of failure to collect a true sample of the data. Present camera systems, excluding the multicrystal camera, can operate without significant data loss at count rates in the 20,000–30,000 cps range. Some cameras will perform better than others at higher counting rates, but at this time, single pass studies are the only type likely to require such high count rates. Before ordering and relying on the results of first pass radionuclide angiograms, the clinician may wish to discuss the limitation of the camera with the nuclear medicine physician in his or her hospital (Grenier, Bender, et al., 1968).

Collimators

An integral part of the imaging process is the use of collimation to select only the gamma radiation directed parallel to collimator septa. Collimator design takes into account the energy levels of the radionuclides to be used and whether the field of view can be minified or magnified. The availability of special collimators, such as slant-hole or seven-pinhole, along with the appropriate software, allowed early development of tomographic imaging. These collimators have largely been withdrawn from clinical use.

Current cardiac imaging uses low-energy radionuclides. Long and thick septa within the collimator, required for high-energy nuclides, are unnecessary, thus significantly reducing collimator weight. In general, longer septa allow for improved resolution but at the cost of diminished sensitivity. With shorter septa, resolution is diminished and sensitivity is increased. Collimator use is determined on the basis of clinical judgment. Usually a gated nuclear angiogram requires counts rather than resolution, and a high-sensitivity or general-purpose collimator is chosen. For thallium imaging, resolution rather than sensitivity is selected, and a general-purpose or high-resolution collimator is used. For most cardiac imaging, a parallel-hole collimator will be used to minimize geometric distortion. Collimators with septa drilled so that they converge on a focus outside the camera head (converging) or at a point within the camera head (diverging) are also available. The former allow improved image resolution and sensitivity, at the expense of image field size and geometric distortion. The latter provide a larger field of view, but resolution is reduced and geometric distortion increased. Diverging collimators are used for lung scanning when only a small field of view camera is available. The increasing use of larger field of view cameras tends to minimize the requirements for these collimators. Converging collimators may be used for thallium imaging, but this leads to problems in quantification of images (Figure 1-4).

THE COMPUTER

For even routine cardiac imaging, some form of data processing equipment must be immediately at hand. A number of computer systems are available today, and their operation requires varying degrees of expertise. All digital computing devices, however, have two major aspects, hardware (Cradduck, 1976) and software (Lieberman, 1977).

In considering the hardware aspects of a computing system, one must remember that the usual output from a gamma camera consists of X and Y analog signals that relate to the position of the recorded gamma ray. A third or Z signal allows acceptance of the pulse by the camera and computer, and is usually a function of gamma ray energy. In dual isotope studies, Z-A and Z-B signals are generated.

Since they are analog signals, X and Y must be converted to digital (binary) values for computer manipulation. An analog-to-digital converter (ADC) is the electric component of the nuclear medicine computer that performs this function. The time needed for this conversion depends on the degree of resolution required for a digital study. For example, data collection into a 256×256 matrix demands that both the X and Y signals be divided into 256 levels ($256 = 2^8$; i.e., an 8-bit conversion is required for each signal), while a 32×32 matrix needs only 32 levels of division for each X and Y signal ($32 = 2^5$; i.e., a 5-bit conversion is required for each signal). Most ADCs in current use provide at least a 7-bit conversion, which can occur in the order of 1–2 U/second for each X and Y signal. Thus, a theoretical maximum count rate for such an ADC would be 500,000 to $1 \times 10(6)$ cps. This is far in excess of the rate required for clinical studies. After the ADCs have been processed, the information

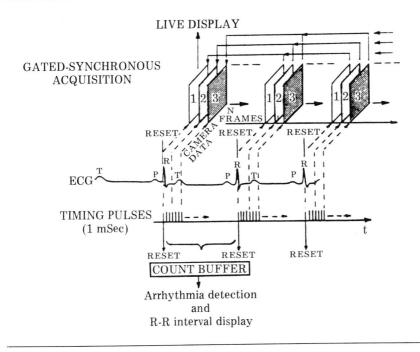

LIVE DISPLAY

GATED-SYNCHRONOUS
ACQUISITION

N
FRAMES

RESET   RESET   RESET

CAMERA
DATA

ECG

TIMING PULSES
(1 mSec)

t

RESET   RESET   RESET

COUNT BUFFER

Arrhythmia detection
and
R-R interval display

Figure 1-4 Diagrammatic representation of gated frame mode data acquisition for cardiac studies. Data from the gamma camera are in N frames between each R wave, with the R wave causing the reset to frame 1. The data collected during each heart beat are added to those from the previous beats so that valid statistical images result. A continuously updated display of the first frame, together with R-R interval, number of cycles collected, and number of cycles rejected, is shown on the computer display screen. (Reproduced, with permission, from Cradduck, T. D. 1981. Computer science. In *Nuclear medicine technology and techniques*, edited by D. R. Bernier, J. K. Langan, and L. Wells, 208. St. Louis: C. V. Mosby.)

is passed directly to and stored in the computer memory.

Before a study is begun, a predetermined matrix size is set up in the memory of the central processing unit (CPU). This matrix will usually be 64 × 64, 128 × 128, or 256 × 256. The choice of matrix size depends on the memory size of the computer and desired resolution. For example, a 128 × 128 matrix provides twice the resolution of a 64 × 64 matrix but requires four times the memory storage capacity. For radionuclide angiography and thallium imaging, a 128 × 128 matrix would be appropriate; this provides a 5 cm resolution with a 300 mm field of view camera, for example, a small field of view mobile camera.

Static images, such as thallium-201 studies, are generally collected to provide maximum resolution with high count accumulations. Dynamic images, such as radionuclide angiograms, are usually time-restricted and do not allow high count collections. Depending on what is clinically appropriate, the nuclear medicine physician or nuclear cardiologist will decide the optimal matrix and acquisition time, both for the particular study and for the available usable memory in the computer. As a rule of thumb, a nuclear cardiology computer should have a memory capacity of 64K words or more. [A "word" usually means 16 bits, or 2^{16}, of memory and equals two bytes (2^8).]

After static or dynamic imaging, data are transferred to a storage device, such as magnetic tape, hard disc, or floppy disc, at the end of collection time. Work load and study type determine the disc storage capacity needed. For example, a thallium study composed of four views collected in a 64×64 word mode will occupy 16K words of memory, while a gated nuclear angiogram requiring three levels of exercise plus a rest study may require 480K words of storage. The capacity of mass storage devices such as discs varies from 500K to more than 100,000K words. Many nuclear cardiology laboratories use these large-capacity discs for immediate day-to-day access of studies and magnetic tape for long-term storage.

Numerous displays and terminals are available, but discussion of this equipment is beyond the scope of this chapter. Displays and terminals are usually part of the computer system and purchased to run with a particular nuclear medicine package.

Although computer hardware is a major consideration, the software, programs needed to perform and analyze nuclear medicine studies, is even more important. There is little point in owning a high-quality computer system that is limited by its processing capabilities. In general, software is composed of an operating system with high-level language compilers (Lieberman, 1977) and application programs (Eason, 1974).

As the name implies, the operating system is composed of a set of programs that allows the computer to function. Application programs, such as those for ejection fraction determination, are said to run "under" the operating system or in conjunction with it. These programs are usually provided by the vendor and are regularly upgraded, but may be modified in-house if special computer expertise is available. In general, reliance is placed on prewritten software (programs), and the quality of this software plays a major role in determining the clinical utility of the computer system.

RADIOPHARMACEUTICALS

Blood Pool Agents

Red blood cells labeled with technetium-99m are currently used as the blood pool imaging agent (Pavel, Zimmer, et al., 1977). Technetium-99m is readily available from molybdenum-99 generators, routinely maintained in nuclear medicine departments, and except for minor restrictions, can be supplied on demand. It has a physical half-life of six hours and a gamma emission of 140 kev. Because of these properties and its ability to be incorporated into many pharmaceutical materials (Castronovo, 1975), technetium-99m is a widely used radionuclide.

The labeling of red blood cells initially involved an in vitro maneuver, with attendant problems of maintaining sterility. Now it is usually done as in vivo labeling, in which a tin-pyrophosphate complex is introduced 15 to 20 minutes before the introduction of the technetium. The tin-pyrophosphate attaches to the red cells, making them more receptive to attachment of technetium. Recent blood transfusions or albumin infusions may interfere with this method.

Thallium

The rationale for using ionic thallium (Tl^+) as a myocardial imaging agent is that it appears to act in a manner similar to ionic potassium (K^+) and rapidly accumulates in living cells (Mullins and Moore, 1960). The radionuclide in current use is thallium-201, introduced in 1975 as a myocardial agent (Lebowitz, Greene, et al., 1975); other isotopes of thallium, such as thallium-199, had been suggested as early as 1970. Transport of thallium across the cell membrane appears to be related to the $Na^+:K^+$ pump and is ATPase-dependent (Gehring and Hammond, 1967). As a result, its accumulation depends on cellular viability as well as on the blood flow carrying it to the area or organ of interest.

Thallium is prepared by cyclotron proton bombardment techniques of thallium-203, to form lead-201, which then decays to thallium-201. Because the process is relatively difficult, thallium-201 is expensive. It decays with a physical half-life of 73 hours, with mercury X-ray peaks in the 67–80 kev range and two lesser peaks at 110 and 160 kev. For imaging purposes, the gamma camera is peaked at 80 kev and a window of 20% to 25% usually set at this photo peak. If dual nuclide facilities are available, the use of the upper peak leads to an increase in the amount of photon flux (counts) detected.

Thallium imaging is best performed using a scintillation camera with an intrinsic resolution of at least 4 mm as measured by a bar phantom at 140 kev, with a general-purpose or high-resolution collimator. One must remember that gamma camera response is significantly worse at 80 kev than at 140 kev, so what can be visualized with technetium cannot necessarily be seen at 80 kev.

Technetium Pyrophosphate

Infarct avid imaging utilizes a technetium pyrophosphate, polyphosphate, or diphosphate derivative. The latter is not generally recommended, since its bone avidity is sufficiently great that rib uptake causes difficulties in scan interpretation of the myocardium.

TECHNIQUES

Associated hardware required for cardiac studies includes ECG gating and monitoring equipment, an exercise bicycle or treadmill, and a defibrillator. The ECG gate and monitor are usually incorporated in a single functional unit. Most available equipment allows the selection of any part of the ECG for triggering the computer. Usually the up-slope of the R wave is chosen to correlate with the end-diastole. Since the actual ECG signal is inappropriate for controlling the computer, a preselected point on the ECG signal generates a simple square wave in another circuit (ECG gate), which is used to trigger the computer.

For ECG monitoring, the standard leads are applied. Lead II is often chosen as the monitor signal. Accurate and firm application of leads is critical to maintain a steady isoelectric line. A varying ECG trace can result in artefactual and erroneous triggering of the ECG gate.

The exercise bicycle used for gated nuclear angiography is generally supplied with a calibrated ergometer. This procedure is often performed in the supine position, although models are now available for semi-erect and upright angiography. The bicycle should have a mechanical configuration that allows patients to exercise easily, without interference from the gamma camera. Sometimes the mechanical design of the camera is such that it does not allow thigh movement during bicycle exercise.

The method of introducing the radiopharmaceutical is critical if a first pass study is to be performed. A "tight" bolus is essential. Introduction via the external jugular vein in infants, or a large medial arm vein in children and adults, is mandatory. Injection into lateral arm veins often leads to delay at venous valves and a stretching out of the bolus. One recommended technique is to use a blood pressure cuff inflated beyond systolic pressure. The sodium pertechnetate is injected, the cuff quickly released, and the arm raised. The study is collected on the computer, and it is then possible to analyze the results on a beat-by-beat basis. Visualization of the cardiac chambers is generally good with this technique, and it has the advantage of "temporal" separation of the right and left ventricles for accurate assessment of ejection fraction wall motion. This technique is particularly useful in shunt detection and assessment of transit time.

The study can be performed with the patient in the right anterior oblique, anterior, or left anterior oblique position, and is usually collected for 20 to 30 seconds, allowing tracing of the movement of the bolus through the right side of the heart, the lung, and into the left side of the heart. It is evident that the total number of counts collected with this technique will be a limiting factor, so a highly sensitive gamma camera (optimally a multicrystal type) will be needed (Cradduck and MacIntyre, 1977).

Techniques of analysis are legion. Most commonly, the data are summed to allow optimal outlining of the left ventricle, either interactively by an operator or automatically. Subsequently, a volume-time curve can be used to obtain end-diastolic and end-systolic peaks. Since we are watching the passage of the bolus through the heart during its first pass, there is no significant background activity. The time-activity curve will have a sinusoidal morphology with peaks and troughs, and these relate directly to end-diastole and end-systole, respectively. Determining the ejection fraction at each beat from these data is fairly simple. The fraction will, in fact, vary from beat to beat, and it is easy to obtain an average ejection fraction. The major advantage of this technique is that background activity does not surround or overlay the left ventricle. One disadvantage is that it is (as the name indicates) a first pass study, so if the clinician wishes to measure ejection fractions at different levels of stress or as a result of interventions, further doses of radioactivity are required. In this context, gated equilibrium studies do not require administration of additional radionuclides. As can be expected, data obtained by both these techniques are quite comparable, and the physician's preference will determine which technique is used. Both techniques correlate well with contrast angiographic determination of ejection fractions and segmental wall motion.

When gated equilibrium studies (Strauss, McKusick, et al., 1979) are performed, the rapidity with which the pertechnetate is introduced is not critical, but the degree of labeling to red blood cells is. With pertechnetate, a number of techniques are used to optimize in vivo labeling. One involves inserting a butterfly needle (21 gauge) with a three-way stopcock into a medial cubital vein. A syringe containing 10 mL of normal saline is inserted into one outlet of the stopcock and blood is withdrawn into a second syringe containing the pertechnetate, via another outlet. The sphygmomanometer cuff is blown up above systolic pressure, and the blood in the pertechnetate syringe is reinjected into the arm through the butterfly needle. The pertechnetate is followed by the saline, after which the cuff is released. If the blood is allowed to remain in the pertechnetate syringe for a minute or two prior to injection, labeling is generally improved.

The gated cardiac blood pool scans have been found useful in determining ejection fraction and qualitatively evaluating regional wall motion. These studies are limited by the superimposition of cardiac chambers in some views and the requirement for long acquisition time and a stable cardiac rhythm. On the other hand, repeat acquisitions in multiple projections, or studies before, during, and after an intervention such as exercise can be acquired for one to two hours with one dose of radiation (to be discussed in greater detail in Chapter 7).

Technetium pyrophosphate (Tc-PYP), usually given in a dose of 10–15 mci intravenously for acute infarct imaging, is thought to bind through phosphate complexes to ionic calcium. This radionuclide was originally introduced as a bone scanning agent, but since local transient increases in Ca^{2+} appear to exist in infarcted or severely ischemic tissue (Willerson, Parkey, et al., 1980), the Tc-PYP was found to accumulate in such tissues.

The rate of accumulation is somewhat faster; imaging requiring three to six hours for bone can be performed within one hour in the case of infarcts. In contrast to thallium, Tc-PYP accumulates in pathological myocardial tissue, and infarcts or aneurysms appear as "hot areas" of increased activity. This imaging is usually performed in the anterior, 45° left anterior oblique, left, and 45° right anterior oblique positions, about 45 to 60 minutes after injection, with a high-resolution collimator. The technique of performing exercise thallium-201 studies is discussed in Chapter 4.

IMAGE PROCESSING AND DISPLAY

Once the camera and the collimator have been selected, a decision must be made concerning the input and recording of data. For most cardiac imaging, direct recording will be performed by computer to allow some form of image processing. In practice, nuclear angiography cannot be performed without a computer system. Thallium and technetium imaging can be performed with only direct film recording, but should if possible be carried out with computer acquisition.

Some form of photographic recording device, usually called a multiformatter, is used if it allows control of image position on a film. The two common media are X-ray film and instant developing film. Either single or double emulsion X-ray film can be used. The former allows a smaller film dot size to be recorded and the latter is more light sensitive. For both types, automated film processing equipment must be located near the examining area. Instant developing film does not require processing, but it is usually more expensive. X-ray film is generally considered to provide better image resolution and contrast, although there is often little to choose from between the performance of the two media in this regard. Film selection is therefore a matter of cost and personal preference.

Nuclear Angiograms

A number of functional parameters are obtained for nuclear angiograms, including data from both the right and left ventricles and data relating to ejection fraction, ejection rates, wall motion, and stroke volume.

As indicated earlier, a number of available software programs can provide the necessary data without the physician interacting with the computer or understanding the mathematical problems involved. In most cases, the major problems relating to correct analysis involve correct outlining of the ventricular edge(s) and accurate determination of background activity.

The position of the camera head in relation to the patient is critical to computer analysis; it must be possible to separate the ventricles (and atria) from each other. Separation is usually ensured by scanning in the 45° left anterior oblique position with a small degree of caudal tilt. Wall motion of all segments may be better assessed by also viewing the anterior and 70° left anterior oblique projection, but these views are used primarily for subjective interpretation.

Detection of ventricular edge may involve physician interaction with the computer by manually outlining the ventricle, using a joystick or a light pen. The physician can also manually define a restricted area for computer research. There are other fully automatic methods in which no user intervention is required. The mathematical mode of edge detection, which is beyond the scope of this description, is dependent upon the statistical accuracy of the image, that is, the number of counts obtained in each frame of the image—the more counts, the better. Temporal restrictions such as exercise are important limiting factors.

The semiautomatic or automatic edge detection routines will often fail at low data levels that can sometimes be found in an exercise study. In this setting, the physician may have to revert to manual (visual) selection of ventricular outlines. Furthermore, for correct volume-time curves (to obtain ventricular contraction and relaxation rates) each frame of a gated study must be analyzed for the ventricular edge. This edge, of course, changes during the ECG cycle. A number of commercially available computer programs for cardiac analysis do not yet provide this capability and use only the end-diastolic outline to calculate these curves. The physician should always be aware of the limitations of the software being used.

Because the radiopharmaceuticals are blood pool agents, they remain in the vascular compartment. Activity seen from the ventricles will be complemented by that from adjacent soft tissues, and in most situations will account for 30% to 40% of the activity seen from the ventricular chamber, so it is essential to correct for this activity before calculating such parameters as the ejection fraction. There is no simple way to correct for background, since it is not constant. A generally useful and relatively accurate technique is to select an area adjacent to the ventricular wall and assume that this is representative of background. Single pass studies do not present this problem, although they do suffer from a general lack of data if performed on an Anger-type camera and not a multicrystal one (Pfizer and Pokropek, 1974).

Difficulties may be encountered if a varying R-R interval (as in sinus arrhythmia), an increasing pulse rate (due to exercise), and ventricular premature beats occur during the study, because the time-activity curve may fail to discriminate the end-systolic frame. The worst situation is usually found in atrial fibrillation. More sophisticated computer processing systems can overcome this or allow arrhythmia analysis during data collection. In practice, the presence of arrhythmias often leads to incorrect analysis of studies; this should be a relative contraindication if only the usual commercial software packages are available or if the user is uncertain of the limitations of the software.

More recent software has led to the development of stroke volume, ejection fraction (Maddox, Holmes, et al., 1978), and phase analysis images. The last is a map of the times of ventricular contraction after the onset of electrical activity. This technique allows functional assessment of conduction abnormalities, better separation of atria and ventricles because of their different contraction rates, and so forth. The clinical usefulness of these parameters remains to be assessed.

Acute Infarct Imaging

Image processing of infarct avid scans usually involves some form of background correction and filtering of rib activity. A number of programs are available for these purposes, but the physician should ensure that computer-generated artefacts are not introduced. Removal of excess background or inappropriate application of smoothing/filtering functions may lead to the introduction of artefacts. If high-quality analog images are obtained simultaneously with the digital images and if he or she is careful not to overprocess the data, the physician is less likely to be misled by the effects of inappropriate digital processing.

Thallium Imaging

As indicated earlier, the collection of thallium-201 imaging data often involves a digital computer. The data are usually collected in static mode in a 64×64 or 128×128 matrix format. Analysis of the data involves one or more different techniques.

One common technique calls for the application of some form of background correction or subtraction to correct the image for background, leaving an image that represents uptake only within the myocardium. Another technique described by Goris, Daspit, et al. (1976) involves circumscribing the ventricular myocardium by a rectangle. The computer is then able to calculate the background activity, using a method of bilinear interpolation at different points in the plane of the rectangle, and to correct this activity; the result is an improved image. Other techniques to correct for the level of background activity include the removal of a fixed percentage of the total activity, and smoothing and applying various filtering algorithms to the image.

All these techniques are subject to various errors, usually due to over- or undercorrection of data. If one wishes to choose a particular technique, it is important to develop a normal set of results to determine whether abnormalities found in later images are artefactual.

Two common techniques have been used for further data analysis of thallium images. One involves clock-type analysis of data (Meade, Bamrah, et al., 1978). The center of the left ventricle is determined manually or automatically, and the counts distributed in the ventricular myocardium are then plotted out as a function of rotation around the myocardium. A method used with commercial software involves clockwise rotation beginning at the 3-o'clock position ($0°$) corresponding to the posterolateral wall on the $45°$ left anterior oblique view and moving through the inferior wall $(90°)$, septum $(180°)$, and base $(270°)$. Using this technique, the physician can determine series of normals and then use these data to determine statistically whether subsequent scans show quantitative abnormalities.

Another technique calls for drawing horizontal or vertical lines through the image as it is shown on the video display and obtaining a plot of activity as a function of distance traversed across the image. The sets of normal data thus obtained can be used to determine whether further data are abnormal.

Both of these techniques allow data comparison of rest and exercise studies and also make it possible to determine in the clockwise manner or in the horizontal or vertical plots whether changes in uptake in the myocardium are significant. A physician who uses these techniques must assume that a significant rotational or translational movement of the heart has not occurred in the interval between the performance of the exercise and rest studies. Thus, very careful attention must be paid to the positioning of the patient and of the camera.

The thallium study can be collected in a gated mode (Hamilton, Narahara, et al., 1978). However, restrictions from relatively low count rates do not allow division of the R-R interval into more than four or five sections if more than 100 to 150K counts per frame are expected and if imaging is to be completed in the appropriate time. In practice, this mode allows collection in one view only since the time for collection, approximately 30 minutes, is not clinically useful.

The most recent innovation is single photon emission computed tomography (SPECT). A number of single photon gamma emission computerized tomographic camera systems (Budinger, 1980) became available in late 1980 and early 1981. In terms of computer reconstruction algorithms, these systems operate similarly to X-ray computerized tomographs (Hounsfield, 1973). This technique employs a rotating gamma camera that allows either $180°$ or $360°$ rotation around the patient. For thallium images, the $180°$ rotation from a right anterior oblique to a left posterior oblique position is often recommended. Experience at the Cleveland Clinic (MacIntyre, Go, et al., 1983) suggests that the $360°$ rotation provides more accurate results despite some theoretical objections to improper attenuation corrections and possible image distortion. Reconstruction algorithms, promoted by commercial software companies, allow "slices" to be developed at various levels of the myocardium. These slices can be manipulated by the computer to form images that would have required other projections. Setting up and performing this type of study demand greater care than standard imaging. Performance is also dependent upon the accuracy of the software. Each institution must determine its own normal results before embarking on pathological diagnosis. It remains to be seen whether this technique will offer a significant diagnostic advantage over the standard nonrotating planar technique.

SPECT imaging of gated studies is technically possible, but involves significant technical, software, and hardware problems, and requires considerable time for adequate data collection. If the R-R interval is to be divided into "n" segments, then "n" sets of data (or rotations) would need to be collected synchronously with each part of the R-R interval. This type of SPECT imaging can be performed with rest studies but not at stress. It appears that SPECT thallium imaging does offer significant diagnostic advantages over the standard nonrotating planar techniques.

References

Ashburn, W. L.; Schelbert, H. R.; and Verba, J. W. 1978. Left ventricular ejection—a review of several radionuclide approaches using the scintillation camera. *Prog. Cardiovasc. Dis.* 20:267–84.

Budinger, T. F. 1980. Physical attributes of single photon tomography. *J. Nucl. Med.* 21:579–92.

Castronovo, F. P., Jr. 1975. Technetium 99m: Basic nuclear physics and chemical properties. *Am. J. Hosp. Pharm.* 32:480–88.

Cradduck, T. D. 1976. Computers in nuclear medicine, part 1. *Appl. Radiol. Nucl. Med.* 5:153–58, 168–70.

Cradduck, T. D.; and MacIntyre, W. J. 1977. Camera-computer systems for rapid dynamic imaging studies. *Semin. Nucl. Med.* 7:323–35.

Eason, C. S. 1974. Computer applications in nuclear medicine. In *Basic science principles in nuclear medicine*, edited by C. M. Boyd and G. V. Dalrymple, 243-58. St. Louis: C. V. Mosby.

Gehring, P. J.; and Hammond, P. B. 1967. The interrelationship between thallium and potassium in animals. *J. Pharmacol. Exp. Ther.* 155:187–201.

Goris, M.; Daspit, S. G.; McLaughlin, P., et al. 1976. Interpolative background subtraction. *J. Nucl. Med.* 17:744–47.

Grenier, R. P.; Bender, M. A.; and Janes, R. H. 1968. A computerized multi-crystal scintillation gamma camera. In *Instrumentation in nuclear medicine*, edited by G. J. Hine, 8-18. New York: Academic Press.

Groch, M. W.; Gottlieb, S.; Mallo, S. M., et al. 1976. A new dual-probe system for the rapid bedside assessment of left ventricular function. *J. Nucl. Med.* 17:930–36.

Hamilton, G. W.; Narahara, K. A.; Trobaugh, G. B., et al. 1978. Thallium-201 myocardial imaging: Characterization of the ECG synchronized images. *J. Nucl. Med.* 19:1103–10.

Hounsfield, G. N. 1973. Computerized transverse axial scanning (tomography). I. Description of system. *Br. J. Radiol.* 46:1016–22.

Lebowitz, E.; Greene, M. Y.; Fairchild, R., et al. 1975. Thallium-201 for medical use, part 1. *J. Nucl. Med.* 16:151–55.

Lieberman, D. E. 1977. *Computer methods.* St. Louis: C. V. Mosby.

MacIntyre, W. J.; Go, R. T.; O'Donnell, J. K., et al. 1983. Personal Communications.

McLaughlin, P.; Coates, G.; and Wood, D. 1975. Detection of acute myocardial infarction by technetium-99m polyphosphate. *Am. J. Cardiol.* 35:390–96.

Maddox, D. E.; Holmes, B. L.; Wynne, J., et al. 1978. Ejection fraction image, a non-invasive index of regional left ventricular wall motion. *Am. J. Cardiol.* 41:1230–38.

Meade, R. C.; Bamrah, V. S.; Hargan, J. D., et al. 1978. Quantitative methods in the evaluation of thallium-201 myocardial perfusion images. *J. Nucl. Med.* 19:1175–78.

Mullins, L. J.; and Moore, R. D. 1960. The movement of thallium ions in muscle. *J. Gen. Physiol.* 43:759–73.

National Electrical Manufacturers Association. 1980. *Performance measurements of scintillation cameras.* Standards publication no. NU 1-1980. Washington, D.C.: National Electrical Manufacturers Association.

Pavel, D. G.; Zimmer, M.; and Patterson, V. N. 1977. In vivo labelling of red blood cells with technetium-99m: A new approach to blood pool visualization. *J. Nucl. Med.* 18:305–08.

Pfizer, S. M.; and Pokropek, T. A. 1974. Processing of noisy functional images. In *Proceedings, first world congress of nuclear medicine*, 161–63 Tokyo: World Federation of Nuclear Medicine and Biology.

Strauss, H. W.; and Pitt, B. 1977. Thallium-201 as a myocardial imaging agent. *Semin. Nucl. Med.* 7:49–58.

Strauss, H. W.; McKusick, K. A.; Boucher, C. A., et al. 1979. Of linens and laces—the eighth anniversary of the gated blood pool scan. *Semin. Nucl. Med.* 9:296–309.

Willerson, J. T.; Parkey, R. W.; Bonte, F. J., et al. 1980. Pathophysiologic considerations and clinicopathologic correlates of technetium-99m stannous pyrophosphate myocardial scintigraphy. *Semin. Nucl. Med.* 10:54–67.

Detection of Acute Myocardial Infarction with Technetium-99m Stannous Pyrophosphate

2

James T. Willerson, M.D.
Robert W. Parkey, M.D.
Samuel E. Lewis, M.D.
L. Maximilian Buja, M.D.
Frederick J. Bonte, M.D.

Department of Internal Medicine
   (Cardiology Division), Radiology, and Pathology
University of Texas Health Science Center
Dallas, Texas

This work was supported by NIH Ischemic SCOR grant no. HL-17669 and by the Harry S. Moss Heart Fund.

Acute myocardial infarction is not always easy to recognize through the use of traditional diagnostic techniques (Eliot and Edwards, 1974; Alison, Moraski, et al., 1975; Roberts, 1976; Poliner, Buja, et al., 1979). Table 2-1 identifies those circumstances in which the clinical recognition of acute myocardial infarction may be difficult. In general, acute myocardial infarcts are difficult to recognize in the presence of left bundle branch block, when several hours or days have elapsed following the onset of chest pain, in those cases in which previous myocardial infarcts have occurred, and/or when myocardial infarction develops during or after open-heart surgery. Enzymatic techniques that are used for the recognition of acute myocardial infarction have temporal limitations. If a patient delays hospital admission for days or even hours after infarction, serial evaluation of cardiac enzymes may miss the event (Shell, Kjekshus, et al., 1971; Roberts, Henry, et al., 1975; Stone, Willerson, et al., 1975; Willerson, Stone, et al., 1977). The capability to localize and ultimately to size the extent of myocardial infarcts is significant, since the prognosis in acute myocardial infarction is related to infarct size (Page, Caulfield, et al., 1971; Roberts, Husain, et al., 1975). Therefore, the development of additional means to identify myocardial infarcts relatively noninvasively, to localize them, and to measure their size provided the original stimulus for the development of technetium-99m stannous pyrophosphate (^{99m}Tc-PYP) myocardial imaging (Bonte, Parkey, et al., 1974; Parkey, Bonte, et al., 1974; Buja, Parkey, et al., 1975; Willerson, Parkey, et al., 1975a, 1975b; Buja, Parkey, et al., 1976; Donsky, Curry, et al., 1976; Parkey, Bonte, et al., 1976; Platt, Mills, et al., 1976; Platt, Parkey, et al., 1976; Pugh, Buja, et al., 1976; Stokely, Buja, et al., 1976; Willerson, Parkey, et al., 1976; Buja, Tofe, et al., 1977; Harford, Weinberg, et al., 1977; Lewis, Buja, et al., 1977; Willerson, Parkey, et al., 1977).

^{99m}Tc-PYP IMAGING IN DETECTION OF ACUTE MYOCARDIAL INFARCTION

The findings of Shen and Jennings (1972) and D'Agostino (1964) suggested that ^{99m}Tc-PYP myocardial imaging could be used to detect acute myocardial infarcts. These investigators demonstrated that calcium is deposited in crystalline form in irreversibly damaged myocardial cells. Bonte, Parkey, et al. (1974) showed that ^{99m}Tc-PYP could be used to detect experimental acute necrosis. Subsequently, extensive studies at our institution and elsewhere have demonstrated that ^{99m}Tc-PYP myocardial imaging can be used to detect the presence of acute myocardial necrosis (Parkey, Bonte, et al., 1974; Buja, Parkey, et al., 1975; Mason, Meyers, et al., 1975; Willerson, Parkey, et al., 1975a, 1975b; Berman, Amsterdam, et al., 1976; Bruno, Cobb, et al., 1976; Buja, Parkey, et al., 1976; Donsky, Curry, et al., 1976; Parkey, Bonte, et al., 1976; Perez, 1976; Platt, Mills, et al., 1976; Platt, Parkey, et al., 1976; Willerson, Parkey, et al., 1976; Zaret, DiCola, et al., 1976; Buja, Poliner, et al., 1977; Buja, Tofe, et al.,

Table 2-1   Clinical circumstances in which recognition of acute myocardial infarcts
may be difficult

Patients with left bundle branch block

Patients delaying their hospital admission for several hours to days after the onset
of symptoms

Patients seen during or after open-heart surgery

Patients who undergo electrical cardioversion

Patients with acute subendocardial myocardial infarcts

Patients with several previous myocardial infarcts

Table 2-2   "Hot spot" radionuclide agents used to detect acute myocardial infarcts

Technetium-99m stannous pyrophosphate

Technetium-99m tetracycline

Technetium-99m glucoheptonate

Anticardiac myosin antibodies

Antimitochondrial antibodies

1977; Lewis, Buja, et al., 1977; Willerson, Parkey, et al., 1977). Other
"hot spot" myocardial imaging techniques have also been used to identify
acute myocardial infarction (Table 2-2) (Holman, Lesch, et al., 1974;
Rossman, Strauss, et al., 1975; Beller, Khaw, et al., 1977; Kulkarni,
Parkey, et al., 1979). Thus far, ^{99m}Tc-PYP has been the most extensively
studied and utilized imaging approach for this purpose.

DETERMINANTS OF ^{99m}Tc-PYP MYOCARDIAL UPTAKE

Studies performed at our institution have identified the three most
important determinants of ^{99m}Tc-PYP myocardial uptake; (a) the presence of myocardial necrosis; (b) residual coronary blood flow of at
least 10% to 40% of control values into the area(s) of irreversible cellular
damage; and (c) the amount of time elapsed following myocardial damage
before ^{99m}Tc-PYP myocardial images are obtained (Parkey, Bonte, et al.,
1974; Buja, Parkey, et al., 1975; Willerson, Parkey, et al., 1975a, 1975b;
Buja, Parkey, et al., 1976; Parkey, Bonte, et al., 1976; Pugh, Buja, et al.,
1976; Willerson, Parkey, et al., 1976; Harford, Weinberg, et al., 1977;
Lewis, Buja, et al., 1977; Willerson, Parkey, et al., 1977).

    We have found in experimental studies that ^{99m}Tc-PYP uptake is
greatest in canine myocardial infarcts produced by permanent coronary
occlusion in which coronary blood flow is reduced to levels of 10% to
40% of control values. If the occlusion is positioned high around the left

anterior descending coronary artery, ^{99m}Tc-PYP uptake is initially reduced in the center of the gross necrosis; the imaging pattern so produced is referred to as the "doughnut" pattern.

Doughnut ^{99m}Tc-PYP images also occur in humans (Figure 2-1) with anterolateral myocardial infarcts. These images are significantly larger than nondoughnut anterolateral lesions. Congestive heart failure often develops in patients with ^{99m}Tc-PYP doughnut lesions (Willerson, Parkey, et al., 1975a; Rude, Parkey, et al., 1979). Patients with doughnut ^{99m}Tc-PYP myocardial images who die typically have either complete occlusion or severe narrowing of the proximal left anterior descending coronary artery and often additional coronary disease as well (Rude, Parkey, et al., 1979).

In experimental animals, when the occlusion is more distal around the left anterior descending coronary artery and/or when collateral flow is large, the doughnut pattern does not occur. Instead, the ^{99m}Tc-PYP myocardial uptake in the region(s) of myocardial necrosis is more homogeneous. In both humans and experimental animals with doughnut patterns, the center of the doughnut often becomes filled in during the first few days following acute myocardial infarction. This filling-in occurs because increases in collateral blood flow reach the more central portions of the infarct and perfuse areas that initially received either no flow or severely reduced coronary flow. These different imaging patterns emphasize that ^{99m}Tc-PYP uptake is dependent upon coronary flow; some flow must reach the area(s) of myocardial damage before increased ^{99m}Tc-PYP myocardial uptake can occur. Fortunately, both in experimental animals and in humans, our empirical observations suggest that in the absence of systemic arterial hypotension almost every myocardial

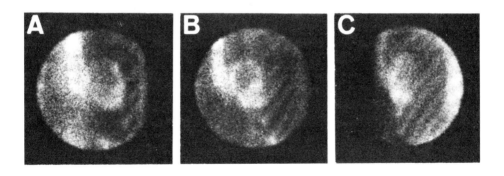

Figure 2-1 A large "doughnut" anterolateral myocardial infarct is shown in the anterior panel (A), left anterior panel (B), and left lateral panel (C) projections. Notice the central defect surrounded by intense ^{99m}Tc-PYP uptake.

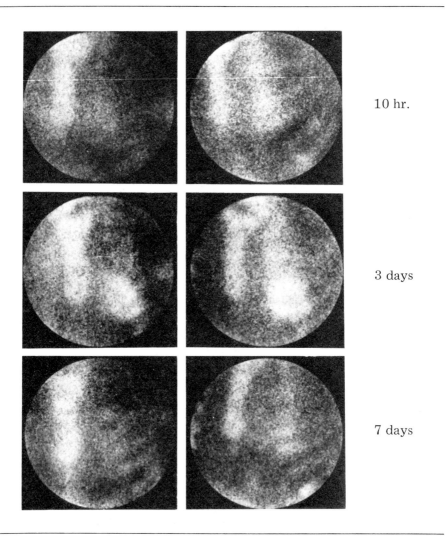

10 hr.

3 days

7 days

Figure 2-2 The serial changes in ^{99m}Tc-PYP myocardial scintigrams that occur between 10 hours and 7 days after acute myocardial infarction. Note that the scintigrams in the top two panels are only faintly abnormal, whereas the ^{99m}Tc-PYP scintigrams are clearly abnormal and demonstrate an apical myocardial infarction. Approximately 7 days after the event, scintigrams are fading and are almost normal.

infarct receives some coronary blood flow, thus allowing the detection of acute myocardial necrosis with this imaging approach (Parkey, Bonte, et al., 1974; Buja, Parkey, et al., 1975; Willerson, Parkey, et al., 1975a, 1975b; Buja, Parkey, et al., 1976; Donsky, Curry, et al., 1976; Parkey, Bonte, et al., 1976; Platt, Mills, et al., 1976; Platt, Parkey, et al., 1976; Pugh, Buja, et al., 1976; Stokely, Buja, et al., 1976; Willerson, Parkey, et al., 1976; Buja, Poliner, et al., 1977; Buja, Tofe, et al., 1977; Harford, Weinberg, et al., 1977; Lewis, Buja, et al., 1977; Willerson, Parkey, et al., 1977; Willerson, Parkey, et al., 1977; Poliner, Buja, et al., 1979; Rude, Parkey, et al., 1979). It should be emphasized, however, that serial myocardial imaging may sometimes be necessary to detect infarction in the occasional patient in whom collateral flow adjustments require longer periods to develop (Falkoff, Parkey, et al., 1978).

Typically, the ^{99m}Tc-PYP myocardial images become abnormal within 10 to 12 hours after the onset of suggestive symptoms, and they become increasingly abnormal in the first 24 to 72 hours after the event (Figure 2-2) (Buja, Parkey, et al., 1975; Willerson, Parkey, et al., 1975b; Buja, Parkey, et al., 1976; Buja, Poliner, et al., 1977; Buja, Tofe, et al., 1977). The development of abnormal ^{99m}Tc-PYP images and their increasing positivity in the first three days following experimental myocardial infarction correlate temporally and topographically with the development and progressive deposition of calcium within the damaged myocardial regions (Buja, Parkey, et al., 1975; Buja, Parkey, et al., 1976). Our experimental studies suggest that ^{99m}Tc-PYP forms a complex with calcium in a subcrystalline or crystalline form in vitro; this binding is not altered by albumin binding to the ^{99m}Tc-PYP (Buja, Tofe, et al., 1977). We have, therefore, proposed that a major mechanism in the ^{99m}Tc-PYP concentration in irreversibly damaged myocardial tissue is the complexing of pyrophosphate to calcium deposited in irreversibly injured cells (Buja, Tofe, et al., 1977).

TRANSMURAL MYOCARDIAL INFARCTS IDENTIFIED BY IMAGING

Figure 2-3 demonstrates the various types of transmural myocardial infarcts identified by ^{99m}Tc-PYP imaging. Unfortunately, many nontransmural infarcts demonstrate fainter uptake of the ^{99m}Tc-PYP and can be either well localized or relatively poorly localized (Willerson, Parkey, et al., 1975a; Poliner, Parkey, et al., 1977; Pulido, Parkey, et al., 1980). Figure 2-4 shows the grading scheme we use to interpret ^{99m}Tc-PYP myocardial images. The majority of acute transmural myocardial infarcts demonstrate a "3–4+" pattern of increased ^{99m}Tc-PYP uptake, whereas approximately 50% of nontransmural infarcts demonstrate "2+" ^{99m}Tc-PYP uptake.

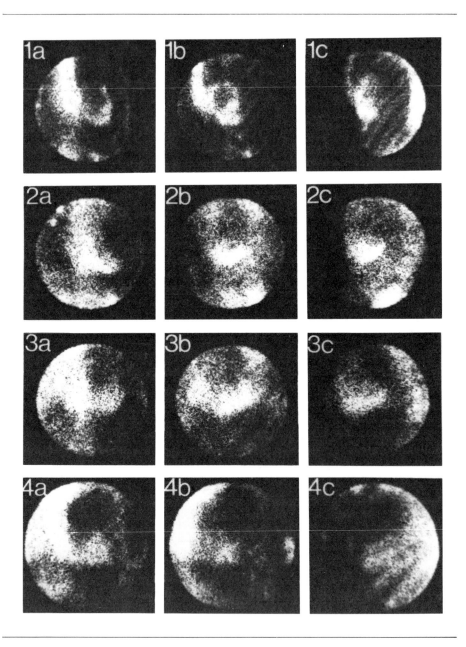

Figure 2-3 The various types of transmural infarcts as demonstrated by ^{99m}Tc-PYP imaging. Panels **A** to **C** in each row represent the anterior, left anterior oblique, and left lateral views. Panels **1A–1C** demonstrate a large antero-lateral myocardial infarct; panels **2A–2C** demonstrate an inferior myocardial infarct; panels **3A–3C** demonstrate an inferolateral and posterior infarct; and panels **4A–4C**, a true posterior myocardial infarction.

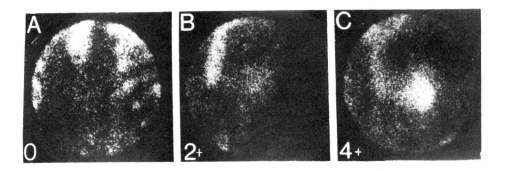

Figure 2-4 The grading scheme used for interpretation of ^{99m}Tc-PYP myocardial scintigrams at our institution. Images that grade from "2+–4+" are
considered abnormal. (See text for details.)

In general, ^{99m}Tc-PYP myocardial imaging has been shown to be
a sensitive and accurate test for the detection of acute myocardial necrosis
(Campeau, Gottlieb, et al., 1975; Ahmad, Dubiel, et al., 1977; Berman,
Amsterdam, et al., 1977; Cowley, Mantle, et al., 1977; Henning, Schelbert, et al., 1977; Olson, Lyons, et al., 1977; Holman, Chisholm, et al.,
1978; Holman, Lesch, et al., 1978; Poliner, Buja, et al., 1979). The evidence includes:

1. Several reported series with a high incidence of abnormal ^{99m}Tc-PYP
    myocardial images in patients with clinical, electrocardiographic, and
    serum enzymatic evidence of acute myocardial infarcts (Mason,
    Myers, et al., 1975; Willerson, Parkey, et al., 1975a, 1975b; Berman,
    Amsterdam, et al., 1976; Bruno, Cobb, et al., 1976; Perez, 1976;
    Zaret, DiCola, et al., 1976; Buja, Tofe, et al., 1977; Willerson, Parkey,
    et al., 1977).

2. Experimental studies showing that selective ^{99m}Tc-PYP concentra-
    tion after acute coronary occlusion is limited to myocardium with
    advanced necrosis or severe damage (Buja, Parkey, et al., 1975;
    Zweiman, Holman, et al., 1975; Buja, Parkey, et al., 1976; Marcus,
    Tomanek, et al., 1976; Buja, Tofe, et al., 1977; Lewis, Buja, et al.,
    1977; Poliner, Buja, et al., 1977; Reimer, Martonffy, et al., 1977).

3. Studies documenting the development of abnormal ^{99m}Tc-PYP
    myocardial images in experimental animals with myocardial necrosis
    induced by conditions other than coronary artery disease and in
    patients with cardioversion-induced myocardial injury and meta-
    static cardiac tumor (Pugh, Buja, et al., 1976; Stokely, Buja, et al.,
    1976; Harford, Weinberg, et al., 1977; McDaniel and Morton, 1977;
    Schneider, Hayslett, et al., 1977).

IMAGING IN DETECTION OF ACUTE MYOCARDIAL NECROSIS

Some observations have raised questions concerning ^{99m}Tc-PYP myocardial imaging for detecting acute myocardial necrosis. These have included the following:

1. The development of low-grade, abnormal ^{99m}Tc-PYP myocardial images in approximately one-third of the patients with unstable angina pectoris, but without electrocardiographic or serum enzyme changes documenting the presence of acute myocardial infarction (Willerson, Parkey, et al., 1975b; Donsky, Curry, et al., 1976).

2. Several reports of a low incidence of abnormal ^{99m}Tc-PYP myocardial images in patients with clinical and laboratory evidence of acute subendocardial myocardial infarction (Karunaratne, Walsh, et al., 1976; Ahmad, Dubiel, et al., 1977; Prasquier, Taradash, et al., 1977).

3. Controversy regarding the importance of "poorly localized" or "diffusely abnormal" images and the difficulty in distinguishing low-grade abnormal from artefactual radionuclide blood pool images (Berman, Amsterdam, et al., 1976; Berman, Amsterdam, et al., 1977; Parkey, Bonte, et al., 1977; Prasquier, Taradash, et al., 1977; Willerson, Parkey, et al., 1977).

4. The development of persistently positive ^{99m}Tc-PYP myocardial images in some patients for weeks to months following acute myocardial infarction without clinical evidence of new infarction (Buja, Poliner, et al., 1977; Olson, Lyons, et al., 1977; Poliner, Buja, et al., 1979).

Clinicopathological Study of 52 Patients

In order to resolve some of these questions, we performed studies that correlated clinicopathological findings in 52 patients who had ^{99m}Tc-PYP myocardial imaging before death or surgical resection of myocardium (Poliner, Buja, et al., 1979). In these 52 patients, 59 clinical events were evaluated; 41 of the 59 were associated with one or more abnormal ^{99m}Tc-PYP myocardial studies and 19 with normal ^{99m}Tc-PYP myocardial images (Poliner, Buja, et al., 1979). In these studies, ^{99m}Tc-PYP myocardial images were abnormal in 29 of 31 patients with clinicopathological evidence of an associated discrete and grossly obvious acute myocardial infarct. Sixteen of 18 acute transmural myocardial infarcts and 13 of 15 subendocardial infarcts were correctly identified during life by the ^{99m}Tc-PYP myocardial images; in the two subendocardial infarcts that were not detected by myocardial imaging, the extent of myocardial damage was estimated to be less than 3 g. In 16 of 18 cases, negative ^{99m}Tc-PYP myocardial images correlated with the absence of acute myocardial infarction as determined by clinicopathological evidence. In two cases, small subendocardial infarcts (less than 3 g) were not detected by ^{99m}Tc-PYP myocardial imaging. Of the 12 additional instances of abnormal ^{99m}Tc-PYP myocardial images, five were associated with clinical evidence of unstable angina pectoris and seven were in individuals with persistently positive myocardial images. In all 12, the abnormal ^{99m}Tc-PYP images were associated with evidence of multifocal irreversible myocardial damage, consisting of myocytolysis, coagulation necrosis, and/or fibrosis; the histological age of the lesions was compatible with acute injury, corresponding to the time of the ^{99m}Tc-PYP myocardial images. Table 2-3 identifies the sensitivity and specificity of ^{99m}Tc-PYP myocardial imaging for the detection of any degree of myocardial necrosis as established by these clinicopathological correlations (Poliner, Buja, et al., 1979). The data obtained in these 52 patients suggest that an abnormal ^{99m}Tc-PYP myocardial image is a sensitive indicator of significant myocardial injury that can manifest itself as gross myocardial necrosis, corresponding to clinical evidence of an acute myocardial infarction, or as multifocal necrosis or myocytolysis associated with unstable angina pectoris or recurrent ischemic heart disease, particularly after previous infarction (Poliner, Buja, et al., 1979).

Certain important technical factors must be adhered to in order to obtain sensitivity and specificity in the detection of myocardial necrosis as defined in the preceding paragraph. Table 2-4 outlines the steps we believe are important in performing the test. To use this test properly, the operator must ensure that the ^{99m}Tc-PYP injectate does not contain an excessive level of ^{99m}Tc-PYP (Stokely, Parkey, et al., 1976; Willerson, Parkey, et al., 1977). If excessive ^{99m}Tc-PYP is present, it can be taken up in red cells, and the result would be a persistent radionuclide blood pool image which could be erroneously interpreted as an abnormal ^{99m}Tc-PYP myocardial image. Of the several methods available for testing ^{99m}Tc-PYP injectate for free ^{99m}Tc-PYP, we use the one shown in Table 2-5.

Table 2-3   Predictive indices for recognition of myocardial necrosis by ^{99m}Tc-PYP myocardial scintigraphy for 59 clinical events in 52 patients

Predictive indices	Microscopic or gross necrosis	Gross myocardial infarct
Prevalence	78%	53%
Sensitivity	89%	94%
Specificity	100%	57%
Predictive value		
Positive scan	100%	71%
Negative scan	72%	98%

Table 2-4   Technical approach to obtaining ^{99m}Tc-PYP myocardial scintigrams

1. Ensure proper labeling of pyrophosphate with ^{99m}Tc-PYP by checking all or representative batches of material for free ^{99m}Tc-PYP.

2. Carefully inject into a vein (not into plastic intravenous [IV] tubing) with good flush.

3. Obtain ^{99m}Tc-PYP myocardial images in at least four projections including the anterior, 35° and 70° left anterior oblique, and left lateral positions. Images are routinely obtained at 2 hours following IV injection, but if there is any question whether a particular image represents a blood pool scintigram, repeat images should be obtained 3 to 4 hours after IV injection. Blood pool scintigrams attributable to delayed renal clearance (severe renal disease, etc.) or severely deranged ventricular function would be expected to clear within that period. However, those attributable to in vivo labeling of red blood cells because of excessive free ^{99m}Tc-PYP in the IV injectate would not clear within that period, and it is necessary to wait until the next day to repeat the test.

4. In positioning the patient and interpreting the ^{99m}Tc-PYP scintigram, it is necessary to be certain that the position of the heart in the chest is known and that the imaging projections will have allowed all of the various myocardial regions to be visualized. In particular, the inferior or diaphragmatic portion of the heart must be well seen.

Table 2-5   Method for testing ^{99m}Tc-PYP for free ^{99m}Tc-pertechnetate

1. Cut silica gel chromatographic paper into 5 × 20 mm strips and dry in desiccator.

2. Place a small drop of ^{99m}Tc-PYP one-half inch from opposite end of paper held with forceps; allow drop to dry in N_2 atmosphere.

3. Set dried paper strip in a bottle with approximately one-quarter inch of methyl-ethyl ketone; drop remains above the level of MEK.

4. After 30 seconds, remove strip and allow it to dry. Then, either image the strip or cut the paper into pieces and count it in a well counter.

5. Discard the ^{99m}Tc-PYP batch if a significant migration of ^{99m}Tc-pertechnetate is detected away from the drop.

IMAGING PATTERNS OF PROGNOSTIC SIGNIFICANCE

Two ^{99m}Tc-PYP myocardial imaging patterns appear to have prognostic significance: the doughnut ^{99m}Tc-PYP images and the persistently positive imaging pattern (Buja, Poliner, et al., 1977; Olson, Lyons, et al., 1977; Poliner, Buja, et al., 1979; Rude, Parkey, et al., 1979). As noted earlier, the doughnut ^{99m}Tc-PYP myocardial images appear when proximal left anterior descending coronary artery occlusion or severe narrowing exists. These images generally identify large anterior or anterolateral myocardial infarcts (Rude, Parkey, et al., 1979). The infarcts tend to be approximately twice as large as nondoughnut anterior or anterolateral infarcts (Rude, Parkey, et al., 1979). Consequently, it comes as no surprise to find that approximately two-thirds of patients with doughnut ^{99m}Tc-PYP myocardial images have a significant degree of congestive heart failure (Rude, Parkey, et al., 1979).

Persistently positive ^{99m}Tc-PYP myocardial images are those that remain abnormal for three months or longer after acute myocardial infarction (Buja, Poliner, et al., 1977). Generally, the ^{99m}Tc-PYP myocardial images become normal approximately six days after myocardial infarction. However, between 10% and 40% of patients with acute myocardial infarcts develop persistently abnormal tests (Buja, Poliner, et al., 1977). Recently, we assessed a series of 40 patients through serial myocardial imaging. Nineteen patients (41%) retained persistently abnormal ^{99m}Tc-PYP myocardial images (usually low-grade "2+" patterns) for at least three months after acute myocardial infarction (Buja, Poliner, et al., 1977). A major clinical difference between patients with persistently abnormal and negative postinfarct ^{99m}Tc-PYP myocardial images was a greater frequency of symptoms after infarction in the group with persistently abnormal tests (Buja, Poliner, et al., 1977). The more symptomatic course consisted of severe angina pectoris in 16 of the 19 patients and severe congestive heart failure with angina in the remaining three. In a separate clinicopathological study of seven patients, persistently abnormal ^{99m}Tc-PYP myocardial images were associated with prominent myocytolytic degeneration involving muscle cells that had survived initial episodes of infarction in five patients (three with ventricular aneurysms) and with extensive myocardial fibrosis in one patient with recurrent angina pectoris. One patient with a negative postinfarct ^{99m}Tc-PYP myocardial image had extensive transmural fibrosis without residual myocardium in a resected ventricular aneurysm. We have suggested that a persistently abnormal ^{99m}Tc-PYP myocardial image frequently correlates with progressive myocardial damage and muscle loss. This pattern may be an important prognostic indicator of a complicated and symptomatic postinfarct clinical course (Buja, Poliner, et al., 1977). Figure 2-5 demonstrates a persistently abnormal ^{99m}Tc-PYP myocardial image. Olson, Lyons, et al. (1977) have also concluded that persistently abnormal ^{99m}Tc-PYP myocardial images have prognostic value and tend to identify those patients who will have persistent and severe angina following myocardial infarction. However, more study is needed to test these relationships further and to establish whether the persistently abnormal ^{99m}Tc-PYP myocardial images are relatively accurate predictors of a poor clinical course after myocardial infarction. If these initial findings are verified, this imaging pattern may serve to identify those patients most at risk of additional ischemic complications early, so that they can be offered more aggressive pharmacological and/or surgical treatment.

9/8/75 4/29/76

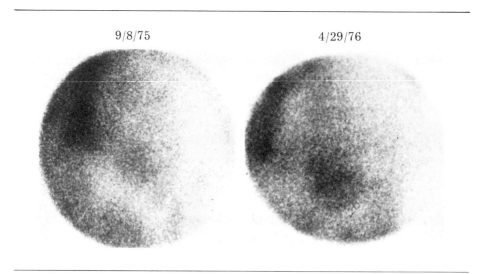

Figure 2-5 A persistently abnormal ^{99m}Tc-PYP myocardial scintigram.

ESTIMATION OF INFARCT SIZE

Through the use of ^{99m}Tc-PYP myocardial imaging, it is possible to accurately size acute anterior or anterolateral transmural infarcts in experimental animals and in humans (Shen and Jennings, 1972; Buja, Tofe, et al., 1977; Willerson, Parkey, et al., 1977). Technetium-99m stannous pyrophosphate myocardial imaging estimates of infarct size in experimental animals with acute anterior or anterolateral infarcts have a close relationship to histologically determined infarct weight (Stokely, Buja, et al., 1976; Buja, Tofe, et al., 1977; Lewis, Buja, et al., 1977: Poliner, Buja, et al., 1977; Willerson, Parkey, et al., 1977). However, it is not yet possible to accurately size acute nontransmural infarcts (subendocardial infarcts) or acute transmural inferior infarcts with currently available imaging equipment. The development of tomographic cameras and three-dimensional image reconstruction techniques will allow accurate estimates of nontransmural and transmural inferior infarct size with gamma emitters (including ^{99m}Tc-PYP).

SUMMARY

Technetium-99m stannous pyrophosphate myocardial images can aid in the detection of acute myocardial necrosis. At least two imaging patterns appear to have prognostic significance in the identification of anatomic findings and/or potential clinical consequences of acute myocardial infarcts. Finally, it is possible to size acute anterior and anterolateral transmural myocardial infarcts with this imaging technique. Tomographic imaging may well make it possible to accurately size almost all infarcts.

References

Ahmad, M.; Dubiel, J. P.; Logan, K. W., et al. 1977. Limited clinical diagnostic specificity of technetium-99m stannous pyrophosphate myocardial imaging in acute myocardial infarction. *Am. J. Cardiol.* 39:50–54.

Alison, H. W.; Moraski, R. E.; Mantle, J. A., et al. 1975. Coronary anatomy and arteriography in patients with unstable angina pectoris. Abstract. *Am. J. Cardiol.* 35:118.

Beller, G. A.; Khaw, B. A.; Haber, E., et al. 1977. Localization of radiolabeled cardiac myosin-specific antibody in myocardial infarcts: Comparison with technetium-99m stannous pyrophosphate. *Circulation* 55:74–78.

Berman, D. S.; Amsterdam, E. A.; Hines, H. H., et al. 1977. New approach to interpretation of technetium-99m pyrophosphate scintigraphy in detection of acute myocardial infarction: Clinical assessment of diagnostic accuracy. *Am. J. Cardiol.* 39:341–46.

Berman, D. S.; Amsterdam, E. A.; Salel, A. F., et al. 1976. Improved diagnostic assessment of acute myocardial infarction: Sensitivity and specificity of Tc-99m pyrophosphate scintigraphy. Abstract, *J. Nucl. Med.* 17:523.

Bonte, F. J.; Parkey, R. W.; Graham, K. D., et al. 1974. A new method for radionuclide imaging of myocardial infarcts. *Radiology* 110:473–74.

Bruno, F. P.; Cobb, F. R.; Rivas, F., et al. 1976. Evaluation of 99m technetium stannous pyrophosphate as an imaging agent in acute myocardial infarction. *Circulation* 54:74–78.

Buja, L. M.; Parkey, R. W.; Dees, J. H., et al. 1975. Morphologic correlates of technetium-99m stannous pyrophosphate imaging of acute myocardial infarcts in dogs. *Circulation* 52:596–607.

Buja, L. M.; Parkey, R. W.; Stokely, E. M., et al. 1976. Pathophysiology of technetium-99m stannous pyrophosphate and thallium-201 scintigraphy of acute anterior myocardial infarcts in dogs. *J. Clin. Invest.* 57:1508–22.

Buja, L. M.; Poliner, L. R.; Parkey, R. W., et al. 1977. Clinico-pathologic study of persistently positive technetium-99m stannous pyrophosphate myocardial scintigrams and myocytolytic degeneration after acute myocardial infarction. *Circulation* 56:1016–23.

Buja, L. M.; Tofe, A. J.; Kulkarni, P. V., et al. 1977. Sites and mechanisms of localization of technetium-99m phosphorus radiopharmaceuticals in acute myocardial infarcts and other tissues. *J. Clin. Invest.* 60:724–40.

Campeau, R. J.; Gottlieb, S.; Chandarlapaty, S. K. C., et al. 1975. Accuracy of technetium-99m labelled phosphates for detection of acute myocardial infarction. Abstract, *J. Nucl. Med.* 16:518.

Cowley, M. J.; Mantle, J. A.; Rogers, W. J., et al. 1977. Technetium-99m stannous pyrophosphate myocardial scintigraphy: Reliability and limitations in assessment of acute myocardial infarction. *Circulation* 56:192–98.

D'Agostino, A. N. 1964. An electron microscopic study of cardiac necrosis produced by 9a-fluorocortisol and sodium phosphate. *Am. J. Pathol.* 45:633–44.

Donsky, M. S.; Curry, R. C.; Parkey, R. W., et al. 1976. Unstable angina pectoris: Clinical, angiographic, and myocardial scintigraphic observations. *Br. Heart J.* 38:257–63.

Eliot, R. S.; and Edwards, J. E. 1974. Pathology of coronary atherosclerosis and its complications. In *The heart*, edited by J. W. Hurst, 1003–17. New York: McGraw-Hill.

Falkoff, M.; Parkey, R. W.; Bonte, F. J., et al. 1978. Technetium-99m stannous pyrophosphate myocardial scintigraphy: The need for serial imaging to detect myocardial infarcts in patients. *Clin. Cardiol.* 1:163–68.

Harford, W.; Weinberg, M.; Buja, L. M., et al. 1977. Positive technetium-99m stannous pyrophosphate myocardial image in a patient with carcinoma of the lung. *Radiology* 122:747–48.

Henning, H.; Schelbert, H. R.; Righetti, A., et al. 1977. Dual myocardial imaging with technetium-99m pyrophosphate and thallium-201 for detecting, localizing and sizing acute myocardial infarction. *Am. J. Cardiol.* 40:147–55.

Holman, B. L.; Chisholm, R. J.; and Braunwald, E. 1978. The prognostic implications of acute myocardial infarct scintigraphy with 99mTc-pyrophosphate. *Circulation* 57:320–26.

Holman, B. L.; Lesch, M.; and Alpert, J. S. 1978. Myocardial scintigraphy with technetium-99m pyrophosphate during the early phase of acute infarction. *Am. J. Cardiol.* 41:39–42.

Holman, B. L.; Lesch, M.; Zweiman, F. G., et al. 1974. Detection and sizing of acute myocardial infarcts with 99mTc(Sn) tetracycline. *N. Engl. J. Med.* 291:195–263.

Karunaratne, H. B.; Walsh, W. F.; Fill, H. R., et al. 1976. Technetium-99m pyrophosphate myocardial scintigraphy in patients with chest pain: Lack of diagnostic specificity. *J. Nucl. Med.* 17:523.

Kulkarni, P.; Parkey, R.; Buja, L. M., et al. 1979. Localization of antimitochondrial antibody in experimental canine myocardial infarcts. Abstract, *Circulation* 60 (suppl. II):97.

Lewis, M.; Buja, L. M.; Saffer, S., et al. 1977. Experimental infarct sizing utilizing computer processing and a three-dimensional model. *Science* 197:167–69.

McDaniel, M. M.; and Morton, M. E. 1977. 99mTc-pyrophosphate imaging demonstrating skeletal muscle and myocardial activity following cardioversion. *Clin. Nucl. Med.* 2:57–59.

Marcus, M. L.; Tomanek, R. J.; Ehrhardt, J. C., et al. 1976. Relationships between myocardial perfusion, myocardial necrosis and technetium-99m pyrophosphate uptake in dogs subjected to sudden coronary occlusion. *Circulation* 54:647–53.

Mason, J. W.; Myers, R. S.; Kriss, J. P., et al. 1975. Technetium-99m pyrophosphate myocardial scanning in coronary surgery patients. Abstract, *Circulation* 52 (suppl. II):54.

Olson, H. G.; Lyons, K. P.; Aronow, W. S., et al. 1977. Follow-up technetium-99m stannous pyrophosphate myocardial scintigrams after acute myocardial infarction. *Circulation* 56:181–87.

Page, D. L.; Caulfield, J. B.; Kastor, J. A., et al. 1971. Myocardial changes associated with cardiogenic shock. *N. Engl. J. Med.* 285:133–37.

Parkey, R. W.; Bonte, F. J.; Meyer, S. L., et al. 1974. A new method for radionuclide imaging of acute myocardial infarction in humans. *Circulation* 50:540–46.

Parkey, R. W.; Bonte, F. J.; Stokely, E. M., et al. 1976. Acute myocardial infarction imaged with ^{99m}Tc-stannous pyrophosphate and ^{201}T1: A clinical evaluation. *J. Nucl. Med.* 17:771–79.

Perez, L. A. 1976. Clinical experience: Technetium-99m labeled phosphates in myocardial imaging. *Clin. Nucl. Med.*1:2–9.

Platt, M. R.; Mills, L. J.; Parkey, R. W., et al. 1976. Perioperative myocardial infarction diagnosed by technetium-99m stannous pyrophosphate myocardial scintigrams. Abstract, *Circulation* 54 (suppl. III):24.

Platt, M. R.; Parkey, R. W.; Willerson, J. T., et al. 1976. Technetium stannous pyrophosphate myocardial scintigrams in the recognition of myocardial infarction in patients undergoing coronary artery revascularization. *Ann. Thorac. Surg.* 21:311–17.

Poliner, L. R.; Buja, L. M.; Parkey, R. W., et al. 1977. Comparative evaluation of several different noninvasive methods of infarct sizing during experimental myocardial infarction. *J. Nucl. Med.* 18:517–23.

———. 1979. Clinicopathologic findings in 52 patients studied by technetium-99m stannous pyrophosphate myocardial scintigraphy. *Circulation* 59:257–67.

Poliner, L. R.; Parkey, R. W.; Buja, L. M., et al. 1977. Technetium-99m stannous pyrophosphate myocardial scintigraphy in the recognition of acute subendocardial myocardial infarction in patients. *Tex. Med.* 73:74–81.

Prasquier, R.; Taradash, M. R.; Botvinick, E. H., et al. 1977. The specificity of the diffuse pattern of cardiac uptake in myocardial infarction imaging with technetium-99m stannous pyrophosphate. *Circulation* 55:61–66.

Pugh, B. R.; Buja, L. M.; Parkey, R. W., et al. 1976. Cardioversion and "false positive" technetium-99m stannous pyrophosphate myocardial scintigrams. *Circulation* 54:399–403.

Pulido, J. I.; Parkey, R. W.; Lewis, S. E., et al. 1980. Acute subendocardial myocardial infarction: Its detection by technetium-99m stannous pyrophosphate myocardial scintigraphy. *Clin. Nucl. Med.* 5:191–95.

Reimer, K. A.; Martonffy, K.; Schumacher, B. L., et al. 1977. Localization of 99mTc-labeled pyrophosphate and calcium in myocardial infarcts after temporary coronary occlusion in dogs. *Proc. Soc. Exp. Biol. Med.* 156:272–76.

Roberts, R.; Henry, P. D.; and Sobel, B. E. 1975. An improved basis for enzymatic estimation of infarct size. *Circulation* 42:743–54.

Roberts, R.; Husain, A.; Ambos, H. D., et al. 1975. Relation between infarct size and ventricular arrhythmia. *Br. Heart J.* 37:1169–75.

Roberts, W. C. 1976. The coronary arteries and left ventricle in clinically isolated angina pectoris: A necropsy analysis. *Circulation* 54:388–90.

Rossman, D. J.; Strauss, H. W.; Siegel, M. E., et al. 1975. Accumulation of 99mTc-glucoheptonate in acutely infarcted myocardium. *J. Nucl. Med.* 16:875–78.

Rude, R. E.; Parkey, R. W.; Bonte, F. J., et al. 1979. Clinical implications of the technetium-99m stannous pyrophosphate myocardial scintigraphic "doughnut" pattern in patients with acute myocardial infarcts. *Circulation* 59:721–30.

Schneider, R. M.; Hayslett, P. J.; Downing, S. E., et al. 1977. Effect of methylprednisolone upon technetium-99m pyrophosphate assessment of myocardial necrosis in the canine countershock model. *Circulation* 56:1029–34.

Shell, W. E.; Kjekshus, J. K.; and Sobel, B. E. 1971. Quantitative assessment of the extent of myocardial infarction in the conscious dog by means of analysis of serial changes in serum creatine phosphokinase activity. *J. Clin. Invest.* 50:2614–25.

Shen, A. C.; and Jennings, R. B. 1972. Myocardial calcium and magnesium in acute ischemic injury. *Am. J. Pathol.* 67:417–40.

Stokely, E. M.; Buja, L. M.; Lewis, S. E., et al. 1976. Measurement of acute myocardial infarcts in dogs with technetium-99m stannous pyrophosphate scintigrams. *J. Nucl. Med.* 17:1–5.

Stokely, E. M.; Parkey, R. W.; Bonte, F. J., et al. 1976. Gated blood pool imaging following 99mTc stannous pyrophosphate imaging. *Radiology* 120:433–34.

Stone, M. J.; Willerson, J. T.; Gomez-Sanchez, C. E., et al. 1975. Radio-immunoassay of myoglobin in human serum: Results in patients with acute myocardial infarction. *J. Clin. Invest.* 56:1334–39.

Willerson, J. T.; Parkey, R. W.; Bonte, F. J., et al. 1975a. Acute subendo-cardial myocardial infarction in patients: Its detection by technetium-99m stannous pyrophosphate myocardial scintigrams. *Circulation* 51:436–41.

———. 1975b. Technetium-99m stannous pyrophosphate myocardial scintigrams in patients with chest pain of varying etiology. *Circulation* 51:1046–52.

———. 1976. Technetium-99m stannous pyrophosphate myocardial scin-tigraphy: A new method of proven value for the diagnosis and localiza-tion of acute myocardial infarcts and for detection of infarct extension in patients. *Tex. Med.* 72:61–66.

Willerson, J. T.; Parkey, R. W.; Buja, L. M., et al. 1977. Are technetium-99m stannous pyrophosphate myocardial scintigrams clinically useful? *Clin. Nucl. Med.* 2:137–45.

Willerson, J. T.; Parkey, R. W.; Stokely, E. M., et al. 1977. Infarct sizing with technetium-99m stannous pyrophosphate scintigraphy in dogs and man: Relationship between scintigraphic and precordial mapping esti-mates of infarct size in patients. *Cardiovasc. Res.* 11:291–98.

Willerson, J. T.; Stone, M. J.; Ting, R., et al. 1977. Radioimmunoassay of CPK-B isoenzyme in human sera: Results in patients with acute myo-cardial infarction. *Proc. Natl. Acad. Sci. U.S.A.* 71:1711–15.

Zaret, B. L.; DiCola, V. C.; Donabedian, R. K., et al. 1976. Dual radio-nuclide study of myocardial infarction: Relationships between myocardial uptake of potassium-43, technetium-99m stannous pyrophosphate, re-gional myocardial blood flow and creatine phosphokinase depletion. *Circulation* 53:422–28.

Zweiman, F. J.; Holman, B. L.; O'Keefe, A., et al. 1975. Selective uptake of 99mTc complexes and 67Ga in acutely infarcted myocardium. *J. Nucl. Med.* 16:975–79.

3 Assessment of Myocardial Infarction with Thallium-201

Frans J. Wackers, M.D.

Associate Professor of Diagnostic Radiology
   and Medicine
Yale University School of Medicine
New Haven, Connecticut

Thallium-201 (^{201}Tl) scintigraphy performed at the bedside of patients with acute myocardial infarction is a simple and sensitive method for detecting, localizing, and estimating the size of the infarct. In particular, the size of the perfusion defect is of value as a prognostic parameter in patients without heart failure. The high sensitivity of ^{201}Tl scintigraphy for use in the early hours of acute infarction makes it a potentially useful procedure for triage of patients with acute chest pain in the emergency room.

INTERPRETATION OF ^{201}Tl IMAGES

The correct interpretation of ^{201}Tl images in patients with acute myocardial infarction depends upon a thorough understanding of the anatomy of the heart as projected on the different scintigraphic views. In normal subjects in the resting state, only the left ventricle is well visualized (Figure 3-1). The right ventricle, because its myocardial mass is smaller and its accumulation of ^{201}Tl is relatively less per gram of tissue, is usually visualized only faintly, if at all (Wackers, van der Schoot, et al., 1975).

In patients with normal myocardial perfusion, the left ventricle appears to be horseshoe or ovoid in shape. The distribution of ^{201}Tl in the left ventricle is almost homogeneous, although the normal subject may show some areas with slightly diminished uptake. The central area of diminished activity on all views represents the ventricular cavity. Commonly, decreased activity is seen in a small area of the apex; this sign, which is a result of normal thinning of the myocardium in this region, is not abnormal.

Routinely, three views should be obtained to permit a systematic evaluation of the entire myocardium. Furthermore, diagnostic reliability is enhanced when a defect corresponding to a given anatomic location is present in more than one projection. The three important views for myocardial imaging with ^{201}Tl are the $0°$ anterior and $45°$ left anterior oblique (both with the patient supine), and the $90°$ left lateral view (with the patient turned on the right side). The effect of patient positioning (Johnstone, Wackers, et al., 1979) on the ^{201}Tl images in the left lateral projection is illustrated in Figure 3-2. It is important to realize that in many patients a $70°$–$80°$ left anterior oblique supine view is not comparable to the $90°$ left lateral view with the patient on his or her right side. Depending on the position of the heart, the posterior wall may not be visualized or may be seen only incompletely on a steep supine projection. The anatomy of the left ventricle as projected on to various scintigraphic views is shown in Figure 3-3.

In our laboratory we read ^{201}Tl images as positive, questionable, or normal (see Chapter 5 for alternate reading schemes). The judgment concerning diminished or absent regional activity is made qualitatively by comparing ^{201}Tl uptake in different areas of the left ventricle. Positive

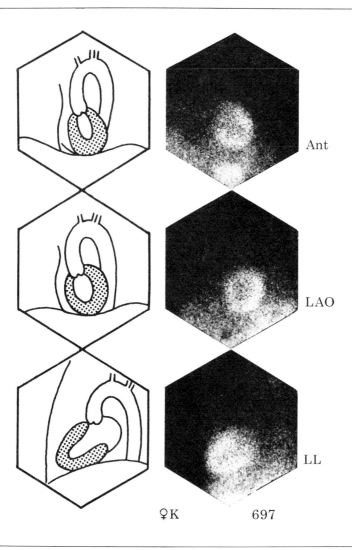

Figure 3-1 Thallium-201 scintiscans of a normal subject. On the left are representations of the anatomy. **Ant**, anterior; **LAO**, left anterior oblique; **LL**, left lateral. (Reproduced, with permission, from Ritchie, J. L.; Hamilton, G. W.; and Wackers, F. J. T., editors. 1978. *Thallium-201 myocardial imaging*, 42. New York: Raven Press.)

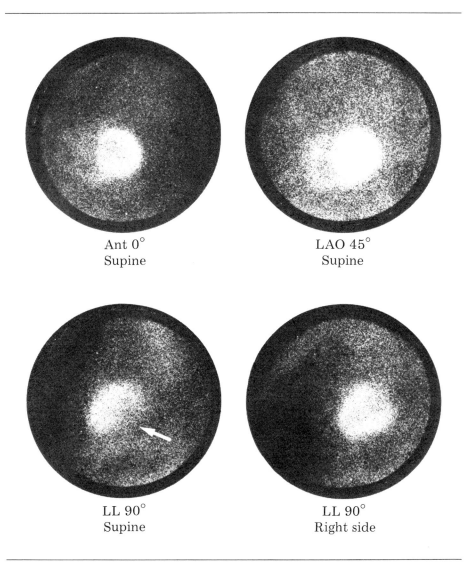

Ant 0°
Supine

LAO 45°
Supine

LL 90°
Supine

LL 90°
Right side

Figure 3-2 Thallium-201 scintigraphy in four projections in a patient with normal coronary arteries. An inferoposterior defect is seen on the **LL** image in the supine position, but is not apparent on the **LL** image with the patient on his right side. The anterior (**Ant**) and 45° **LAO** images (top) are normal. The "defect" on the **LL** supine image is artefactual. (Reproduced, with permission, from Johnstone, D. E.; Wackers, F. J. T.; Berger, H. J., et al. 1979. *J. Nucl. Med.* 20:183-88.)

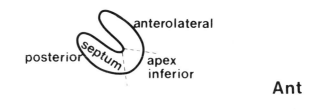

Ant

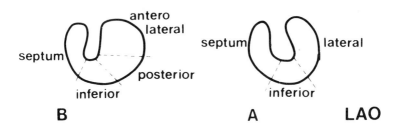

B   **A**   **LAO**

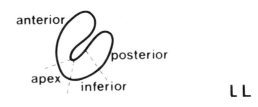

L L

Figure 3-3 Schematic representation of the anatomy of the left ventricle in different scintigraphic views. On the 45° LAO view the posterolateral wall is not always visualized in the same way. In **A** the longitudinal axis of the ventricle is approximately perpendicular to the position of the collimator, whereas in **B** the heart is turned slightly more to the medial line, resulting in a symmetrical image. The asymmetrical image is partly due to motion artefact of cardiac contraction. The posterolateral image moves inwards across the plane of view, resulting in a "blurred" image (Hamilton, Narahara, et al., 1978). The septal movement is perpendicular to the plane of view and the result is a relatively thinner image. (Reproduced, by permission of the American Heart Association Inc., from Wackers, F. J. T.; Becker, A. E.; Samson, G., et al. 1977. *Circulation* 56:72-78.)

images show an anatomically consistent area of definite diminished ^{201}Tl activity equal to or less than lung activity on all three views. Questionable images represent either an anatomically consistent area with diminished activity on all three views or a defect on only one view. Normal images show homogeneous uptake in the left ventricle on all three views.

Recently, computer-generated circumferential count profiles of myocardial distribution of ^{201}Tl have rendered the interpretation of ^{201}Tl images less subjective. The presence or absence of myocardial perfusion defects can now be assessed objectively by comparing the patient's count profile with lower limits of normal ^{201}Tl distribution.

Initially, ^{201}Tl accumulates in the myocardium as a function of regional myocardial blood flow (Strauss, Harrison, et al., 1975; DiCola, Downing, et al., 1977) and the integrity of the Na^+K^+ATPase system (Gelbart, Doherty, et al., 1976). The tracer is cleared from the blood and accumulates in the heart within 5 to 10 minutes of intravenous injection. Thus, myocardial imaging can be started shortly after the radiopharmaceutical is administered.

Myocardial infarction is visualized on ^{201}Tl images as an area of definite diminished activity. The three views routinely taken are usually sufficient to allow accurate determination of the anatomic extent of the perfusion defect.

Infarctions produce typical images at various anatomic locations. Figure 3-4 shows examples of typical ^{201}Tl images in patients with acute myocardial infarction, and Figure 3-5 is a schematic representation of those images. In patients who have died from complications of acute infarction within a few days of ^{201}Tl imaging, the clinicopathologic correlation between the postmortem location of the infarct and the imaging location is better than for the electrocardiographically determined location (Wackers, Becker, et al., 1977). Accurate location of acute myocardial infarction has clinical relevance, since the location has prognostic significance. It is well known that patients with an anterior wall infarction have a poorer prognosis than patients with an inferior wall infarction. Moreover, involvement of the septum in anterior wall infarction is associated with a mortality that is three times higher than in infarction at other locations.

TIME DEPENDENCY OF ^{201}Tl IMAGING

Imaging with ^{201}Tl is highly sensitive in the detection of acute myocardial infarction; however, this sensitivity depends upon the time of imaging after the onset of acute chest pain and, to a lesser extent, on the size of the infarction (Wackers, Sokole, et al., 1976). In a group of 200 patients with a proven acute myocardial infarction the overall sensitivity was 82%. The sensitivity in patients with small infarctions (SGOT less than 3.5 times upper limits of normal) was 57% and in patients with nontransmural

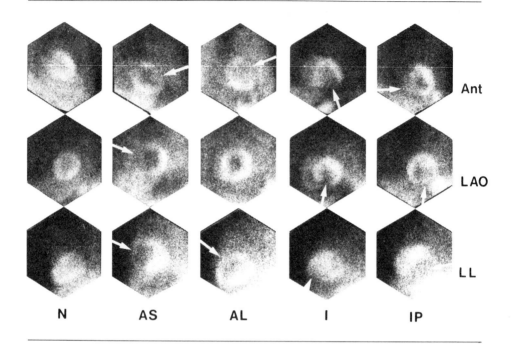

Figure 3-4 Typical scintigraphic images with ^{201}Tl in patients with an anteroseptal (**AS**), anterolateral (**AL**), inferior (**I**), and inferoposterior (**IP**) acute infarction. N, normal subject. (Reproduced, by permission, from the New England
Journal of Medicine [295, 1-5, 1976].)

infarctions (enzyme abnormalities without electrocardiographic Q waves),
63%. Other investigators (Berger, Gottschalk, et al., 1978; Henning,
Schelbert, et al., 1977) have reported a similar degree of sensitivity in the
detection of acute myocardial infarction. A definite relationship existed
between the results of imaging and the time of imaging after onset of
infarction (Figure 3-6). All patients studied early (within six hours) had
definite image defects. Of those studied more than 24 hours after the
onset of symptoms, only 72% had image defects. The results of imaging
were also related to the size of the infarct and whether the infarct was
transmural or nontransmural (Figure 3-7). All patients with large infarctions (peak SGOT more than 3.5 times the upper limit of normal) had
abnormal images throughout the first 24 hours. After that time, some
false negatives (2%) and questionable images (4%) were obtained. Early
(six to 24 hours after infarction) false negatives and questionable images
were obtained only in patients with small or nontransmural infarctions.
    This time dependency of the results of ^{201}Tl imaging in acute myo-
cardial infarction can be explained by the observation that the size of perfusion defects in the same patient often tends to decrease with time. In

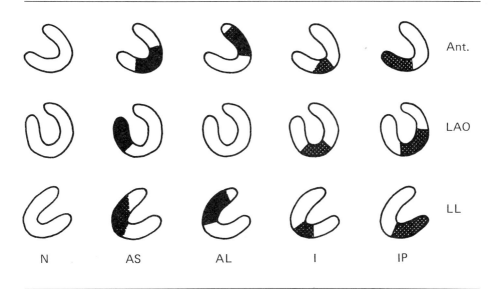

Figure 3-5 Schematic representation of the images in Figure 3-4.

some patients with small infarctions the images may become normal after 24 hours (Figure 3-8). Smitherman, Osborn, et al. (1978) confirmed these observations, using serial imaging after a single dose of ^{201}Tl . A reasonable explanation for this phenomenon is that during the early phase of infarction the method detects the surrounding ischemic zone in addition to visualizing the actual infarct. As the circulation in the ischemic zone improves, the area of necrosis may fall below the resolving power of the imaging system and result in false negative scans. These changes are less obvious in patients with moderate to large infarctions; in these patients, the size of the perfusion defect probably reflects accurately the amount of infarcted myocardium.

EVALUATION OF PATIENTS WITH ACUTE MYOCARDIAL INFARCTION

Since ^{201}Tl myocardial imaging visualizes normal myocardium, ^{201}Tl defects can be expressed as a percentage of total left ventricle. We performed planimetry on the images obtained in vivo and compared the results to postmortem size of infarction (Wackers, Becker, et al., 1977). The linear correlation coefficient for the whole group was 0.75. For infarcts in different locations the correlation coefficient was 0.91 for anterior wall infarcts, 0.97 for inferior wall infarcts, and 0.86 for anteroposterior infarction.

Silverman, Becker, et al. (1979) reported a close correlation between

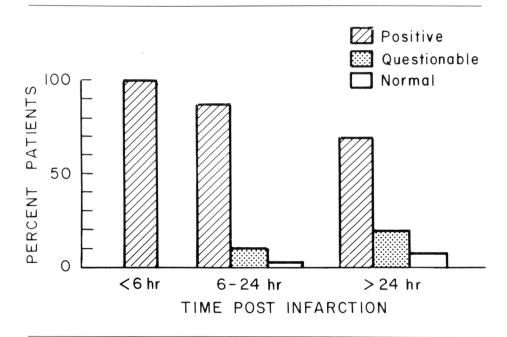

Figure 3-6 Results of ^{201}Tl scintigraphy in 200 patients with acute myocardial infarction in relation to the time after onset of symptoms. (Reproduced, with permission, from Ritchie, J. L.; Hamilton, G. W.; and Wackers, F. J. T., editors. 1978. *Thallium-201 myocardial imaging*, 72. New York: Raven Press.)

the size of the ^{201}Tl defects in stable patients with acute myocardial infarction and their postinfarction course. Large defects correlated highly with early reinfarct and/or death.

Thus, ^{201}Tl imaging may provide an early noninvasive method by which to separate patients with acute myocardial infarction into high-risk and low-risk subgroups. More recently, Perez-Gonzales, Botvinick, et al. (1982) and Botvinick, Perez-Gonzales, et al. (1983) confirmed the late prognostic value of ^{201}Tl defects in patients with and without complicated acute myocardial infarction.

Thallium-201 imaging also proved of value in the evaluation of patients with unstable angina but without infarction (Wackers, Lie, et al., 1978). Imaging performed during the pain-free period after an anginal attack revealed that 40% had perfusion defects. These defects could be distinguished from myocardial infarction, since they showed "filling in" when imaged two to four hours later; apparently the change was a result of redistribution of [201]Tl. The patients with positive images had a higher incidence of complications (acute myocardial infarction or failure to respond to medical treatment, necessitating coronary bypass surgery) than those with negative images.

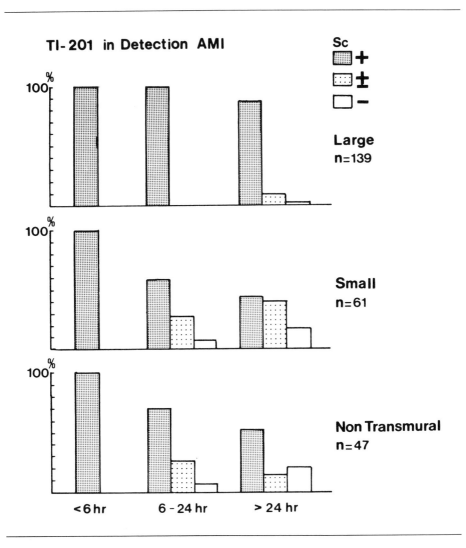

Figure 3-7 Relationship between time of scintigraphy and the extent of acute myocardial infarction. Sc, scintiscans; +, positive; ±, questionable; −, negative or normal. (Reproduced, with permission, from Ritchie, J. L.; Hamilton, G. W.; and Wackers, F. J. T., editors. 1978. *Thallium-201 myocardial imaging*, 73. New York: Raven Press.)

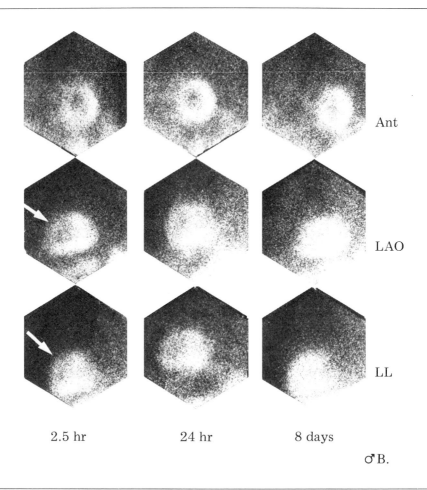

Ant

LAO

LL

2.5 hr   24 hr   8 days

♂ B.

Figure 3-8 Repeated scintigraphy in a patient with a small acute anteroseptal infarction. Arrows indicate a defect at 2.5 hours after the onset of chest pain. At 24 hours the area of diminished activity is still present. Eight days after the onset of symptoms the scintiscans have returned to near normal. (Reproduced, by permission, from the New England Journal of Medicine [295, 1-5, 1976].)

The high sensitivity of ^{201}Tl imaging in detecting acute coronary insufficiency (whether infarction or ischemia) has also proved to be useful in the selection of patients for admission to the coronary care unit (Wackers, Lie, et al., 1979). In many patients the diagnosis of acute myocardial infarction is obvious on their arrival at hospital. However, a significant number are referred to the unit to rule out acute myocardial infarction or ischemia, if the history is questionable and the electrocardiogram nondiagnostic. We studied a group of these highly selected patients by

^{201}Tl imaging at the time of admission, when neither the electrocardiogram nor the history was contributory and the value of ^{201}Tl imaging is maximally challenged. All of the patients who subsequently appeared to have sustained acute myocardial infarction (34 of 203) had abnormal ^{201}Tl images on admission. Definite defects were present in 30 patients, whereas in the remaining four the images were questionable. Positive images were also obtained in 10 of 47 patients who were believed to have unstable angina. Five of these patients and two others who had questionable images progressed to acute myocardial infarction within 24 hours of admission. Positive images were also obtained in nine of 24 patients with previous myocardial infarction.

None of the patients with stable angina and, more importantly, none of the patients who subsequently appeared to have atypical complaints had positive images, although some had questionable ones.

This highly selected subgroup provides a genuine test of the sensitivity, specificity, and predictive accuracy of ^{201}Tl imaging in detecting acute myocardial infarction, and it is this group that needs a reliable selection method. A selection procedure for the coronary care unit or emergency room should be able to detect (a) patients with acute myocardial infarction, (b) patients with unstable angina, and (c) patients with noncardiac complaints. Thallium-201 imaging detects acute myocardial infarction with a sensitivity of 88% and a specificity of 88%, while the predictive accuracy of positive images is 61%. This predictive accuracy is relatively low, owing to positive images obtained in patients with unstable angina and previous myocardial infarction. Lack of specificity is not necessarily a disadvantage, since unstable angina also provides an indication for admission to a coronary care unit. In acute ischemic coronary artery disease a sensitive test is more important than a specific test, since false negative results are less desirable. No false positive images were obtained.

Thallium-201 scintigraphy may make possible a more efficient use of expensive coronary care unit beds. On the basis of history and electrocardiogram alone, 60% of the patients would have been admitted unnecessarily to rule out acute myocardial infarction. When the criterion of admission was positive or questionable ^{201}Tl images, all patients with acute myocardial infarction and the 57% of those with unstable angina would have been admitted. On the other hand, 107 patients would have been allowed to return home, since their ^{201}Tl images were normal. In 87 patients this decision would have been correct and would have avoided unnecessary hospitalization. The remaining 20 patients had "unstable angina" but had an atypical history, a nondiagnostic electrocardiogram, normal images, and an unremarkable and favorable clinical course.

CONCLUSION

Thallium-201 scintigraphy is a sensitive method for detecting acute myocardial infarction, especially during the initial phase. To detect small or nontransmural infarctions, imaging should be performed within 12 to 18 hours of the onset of chest pain.

Thallium-201 imaging allows accurate anatomic location of the infarction and provides a means of estimating the relative size of the malperfused or infarcted myocardium. Important prognostic information can be derived from the size of ^{201}Tl defects in patients without heart failure. In patients with unstable angina, positive ^{201}Tl images indicate a subgroup of patients at higher risk for a complicated clinical course. Another practical application for ^{201}Tl imaging is in patients with an atypical history and nondiagnostic electrocardiogram, in whom it is necessary to rule out acute myocardial infarction.

References

Berger, H. J.; Gottschalk, A.; and Zaret, B. L. 1978. Dual radionuclide study of acute myocardial infarction: Comparison of thallium-201 and technetium-99m stannous pyrophosphate imaging in man. *Ann. Intern. Med.* 88:145-54.

Botvinick, E. H.; Perez-Gonzales, J.; Dunn, R., et al. 1983. Late prognostic value of scintigraphic parameters of acute myocardial infarction size in complicated myocardial infarction without heart failure. *Am. J. Cardiol.* 51:1045–51.

DiCola, V. C.; Downing, S. E.; Donabedian, R. K., et al. 1977. Pathological correlates of thallium-201 myocardial uptake in experimental infarction. *Cardiovasc. Res.* 11:141–46.

Gelbart, A.; Doherty, P. W.; McLaughlin, P., et al. 1976. $Na^+K^+ATPase$ and coronary flow as determinants of thallium-201 uptake by ischemic myocardium. Abstract, *Circulation* 53/54 (suppl. II):70.

Hamilton, G. W.; Narahara, K. A.; Trobaugh, G. B., et al. 1978. Thallium-201 myocardial imaging: Characterization of ECG-synchronized images. *J. Nucl. Med.* 19:1103–10.

Henning, H.; Schelbert, H. R.; Righetti, A., et al. 1977. Dual myocardial imaging with technetium-99m pyrophosphate and thallium-201 for detecting, localizing and sizing acute myocardial infarction. *Am. J. Cardiol.* 40:147–55.

Johnstone, D. E.; Wackers, F. J. T.; Berger, H. J., et al. 1979. Effect of patient positioning on left lateral thallium-201 myocardial images. *J. Nucl. Med.* 20:183–88.

Perez-Gonzales, J.; Botvinick, E. H.; Dunn, R., et al. 1982. The late prognostic value of acute scintigraphic measurement of myocardial infarction size. *Circulation* 66:960–71.

Silverman, K. J.; Becker, L. C.; Bulkley, B. H., et al. 1979. Value of early thallium-201 scintigraphy for predicting mortality in patients with acute myocardial infarction. Abstract, *Clin. Res.* 27:204AA.

Smitherman, T. C.; Osborn, R. C. Jr.; and Narahara, K. A. 1978. Serial myocardial scintigraphy after a single dose of thallium-201 in men after acute myocardial infarction. *Am. J. Cardiol.* 42:177–82.

Strauss, H. W.; Harrison, K.; Langan, J. K., et al. 1975. Thallium-201 for myocardial imaging: Relation of thallium-201 to regional myocardial perfusion. *Circulation* 51:641–45.

Wackers, F. J. T.; Becker, A. E.; Samson, G., et al. 1977. Location and size of acute transmural myocardial infarction estimated from thallium-201 scintiscans. *Circulation* 56:72–78.

Wackers, F. J. T.; Lie, K. I.; Liem, K. L., et al. 1978. Thallium-201 scintigraphy in unstable angina pectoris. *Circulation* 57:738–42.

Wackers, F. J. T.; Lie, K. I.; Liem, K. L., et al. 1979. Potential value of thallium-201 scintigraphy as a means of selecting patients for the coronary care unit. *Br. Heart J.* 41:111–17.

Wackers, F. J. T.; Sokole, E. B.; Samson, G., et al. 1976. Value and limitations of thallium-201 scintigraphy in the acute phase of myocardial infarction. *N. Engl. J. Med.* 295:1–5.

Wackers, F. J. T.; van der Schoot, J. B.; Sokole, E. B., et al. 1975. Noninvasive visualization of acute myocardial infarction in man with thallium-201. *Br. Heart J.* 37:741–44.

4 Mechanism of Angina: Basis for Thallium-201 Myocardial Perfusion Imaging in Coronary Artery Spasm

Graham J. Davies, M.B.
Oberdan Parodi, M.D.
Attilio Maseri, M.D.

Royal Postgraduate Medical School
University of London
London, England

CNR Institute of Clinical Physiology
University of Pisa
Pisa, Italy

Confirmation of acute myocardial ischemia and the investigation of its mechanisms are prerequisites to the logical management of ischemic heart disease. Thallium-201 (^{201}Tl) myocardial perfusion imaging during typical chest pain or acute electrocardiographic changes provides valuable information that is unobtainable from the routine electrocardiogram or coronary arteriogram. A clear understanding of the mechanisms of angina and the theoretical basis for ^{201}Tl imaging is therefore essential.

MECHANISMS OF ANGINA

Effort angina at a constant threshold is probably caused by an increase in myocardial oxygen demand in the presence of a severely limited coronary blood supply, secondary to critical coronary atherosclerotic lesions (Maseri, Severi, Chierchia, et al., 1978). On the other hand, angina at rest with ST segment elevation, as described by Prinzmetal, Kennamer, et al. (1959) and by Prinzmetal, Ekemecki, et al. (1960) has been shown to be caused by coronary vasospasm. Further studies by Maseri, Severi, De Nes, et al. (1978) have demonstrated that a spectrum of disease lies between these two extremes, in which functional changes in coronary flow play a lesser or greater role in the genesis of the anginal attack. Patients can present with angina predominantly at rest or predominantly during exertion. Furthermore, the level of exertion required to induce ischemia may vary considerably from day to day. Attacks of angina in which coronary vasospasm plays a significant part may be associated with ST segment elevation (Maseri, Severi, Chierchia, et al., 1978), depression (Marzilli, L'Abbate, et al., 1977; Maseri, Severi, De Nes, et al., 1978), normalization of previously inverted T waves (Maseri, Severi, De Nes, et al., 1978), or minor changes in the T wave configuration (Maseri, Severi, De Nes, et al., 1978). Apart from the typical rest angina, functional factors affecting the coronary circulation have also been demonstrated during exercise (Specchia, Severi, et al., 1979; Yasue, Omote, et al., 1979) and during cold stimulation (Mudge, Grossman, et al., 1976).

A number of procedures are helpful in deciding which of these mechanisms are operative: (a) history and evaluation of the coronary flow reserve by stress testing (Biagini, Rovai, et al., 1978); (b) provocative tests such as ergometrine maleate injection (Curry, Pepine, et al., 1977); (c) continuous electrocardiographic and hemodynamic monitoring (Maseri, Mimmo, et al., 1975; Chierchia, Brunelli, et al., 1980); (d) coronary arteriography during angina (Dhurandhar, Watt, et al., 1972; Oliva, Potts, et al., 1973; Maseri, Pesola, et al., 1977); and (e) ^{201}Tl myocardial scintigraphy during angina.

THEORETICAL BASIS FOR ^{201}Tl REGIONAL MYOCARDIAL PERFUSION STUDIES

Following intravenous administration, the initial distribution of ^{201}Tl in the heart is proportional to the fraction of the cardiac output perfusing the myocardium. However, for potassium tracers in general, this situation exists only for the time during which a balance is maintained between the amount of tracer not extracted during the first circulation and the amount that re-enters the myocardium on recirculation. This state is achieved only transiently during the initial two minutes and is followed by progressive myocardial uptake for at least 20 minutes (L'Abbate, Biagini, et al., 1979). Ten minutes after injection, arterial ^{201}Tl concentration is reduced to approximately 0.8% and the myocardial uptake is increased by 20%, relative to the level between 20 and 120 seconds (L'Abbate, Biagini, et al., 1979).

The final distribution equilibrium for [201]Tl , as for the other potassium tracers, will tend to be proportional to the potassium pool for the various organs. Therefore, scintigrams recorded shortly after the injection of ^{201}Tl will predominantly reflect regional myocardial perfusion, whereas later images will reflect the distribution of myocardial muscle mass (Maseri, Parodi, et al., 1976). If ischemia is relieved within one or two minutes of ^{201}Tl injection, when the arterial tracer concentration is still high, regional differences in concentration will rapidly disappear because of the high blood-tissue tracer gradient in the ischemic areas. Conversely, when ischemia persists, initial regional differences will be maintained for longer periods.

Regional myocardial perfusion data can be derived from scintigrams recorded five to 20 minutes after injection by comparison with images recorded (a) three or more hours later, when redistribution of the tracer is complete, or (b) several days later, following injection of the same dose of [201]Tl , in the absence of symptoms or acute electrocardiographic changes.

Actual differences in flow between ischemic and nonischemic regions will be underestimated in early scintigrams because potassium tracer clearance is greater at low flow rates (Moir and Debra, 1967; Love, Ishihara, et al., 1968). When the flow is restored before imaging begins, previously ischemic tissue has a larger net extraction than normal tissues. Furthermore, the two-dimensional nature of the images inevitably results in overlap between the ischemic and nonischemic regions, accentuated by the cyclical change in cardiac shape.

The interpretation of transient defects should take into account the following factors:

1. Myocardial uptake, although related to the absolute level of myocardial blood flow, is dependent upon the fraction of cardiac output distributed to the myocardium and surrounding organs and tissues.
2. Ventricular dilatation alone may lead to an apparent extension of areas of decreased activity due to old myocardial infarction.
3. As nonuniformity of tracer distribution occurs in normal subjects, regional differences of less than 20% are probably not significant.
4. Overt ECG changes occur when flow is reduced to 50%–75% of requirements.
5. Over an intermediate range of myocardial blood flow (100-250 mL/min/100 g myocardium), as 100% increase in flow leads to only

a 40% increase in ^{201}Tl uptake (L'Abbate, Biagini, et al., 1979). Thus, massive defects (hardly distinguishable from surrounding background) are most likely caused by a substantial absolute reduction in perfusion (Parodi, Uthurralt, et al., 1981). Massive defects are particularly likely to occur when no increase in heart rate or blood pressure precedes the attack—the most important parameters determining the level of myocardial oxygen demand.

ANGINA AT REST

In a study of 40 patients with spontaneous attacks of angina at rest, we found that ^{201}Tl scintigraphy is invariably positive in the presence of ST segment elevation (Figures 4-1 and 4-2) or with normalization of previously negative T waves (Figures 4-3 and 4-4). The defects are well defined and transmural in nature, and are usually associated with transient complete occlusion of a major coronary vessel, either in the presence or in the absence of underlying atherosclerotic coronary stenosis (Parodi, Uthurralt, et al., 1981). The site of the perfusion defect corresponds to that of the ST segment or T wave changes in the ECG. In the presence of ST segment depression at rest, 95% of patients developed scintigram defects (Figures 4-5 and 4-6). The defects were less well defined than in the case of ST segment elevation or T wave normalization, indicating nontransmural and less severe ischemias. Such patients often have more severe atherosclerotic coronary disease with collateral vessels (Maseri, Severi, De Nes, et al., 1978), and coronary artery spasm seen in these cases is often less extensive or subocclusive (Marzilli, L'Abbate, et al., 1977).

The development of such scintigraphic defects, in the absence of changes indicating an increase in myocardial oxygen demand such as tachycardia or elevation of arterial pressure, strongly suggests a primary reduction of blood supply as the cause of the anginal attack. Coronary arteriography often indicates that this reduced supply is due to arterial spasm.

EFFORT ANGINA

In a study of 58 patients with effort-induced angina, we almost invariably found positive scintigrams in the presence of ST elevation (Figures 4-7 and 4-8) or normalization of T waves (Figures 4-9 and 4-10). Some of these patients also had attacks of angina at rest, and it is therefore probable that an absolute reduction in perfusion is partly responsible for the ischemia. Indeed, coronary artery spasm has been demonstrated by arteriography in some patients with exercise-induced ST segment elevation. As in rest angina, the site of the defect corresponds to the location of the acute ECG changes, and a major vessel is usually involved.

Effort angina with ST segment depression is often associated with normal scintigrams (Figures 4-11 and 4-12). In our series, only 53% of scintigrams were positive.

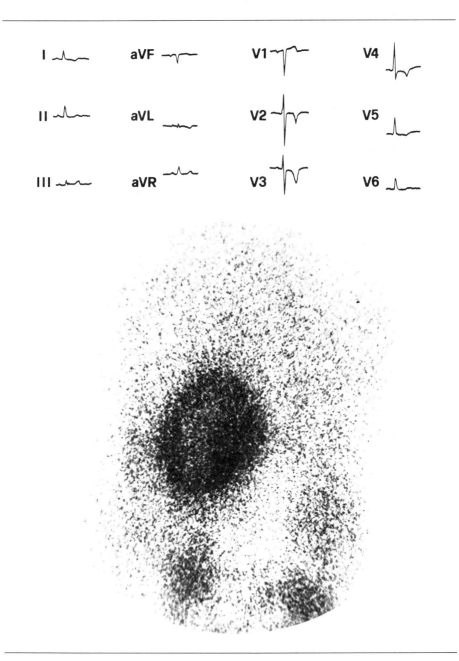

Figure 4-1 ECG and left anterior oblique scintigram recorded in the basal state in a patient with Prinzmetal's variant angina.

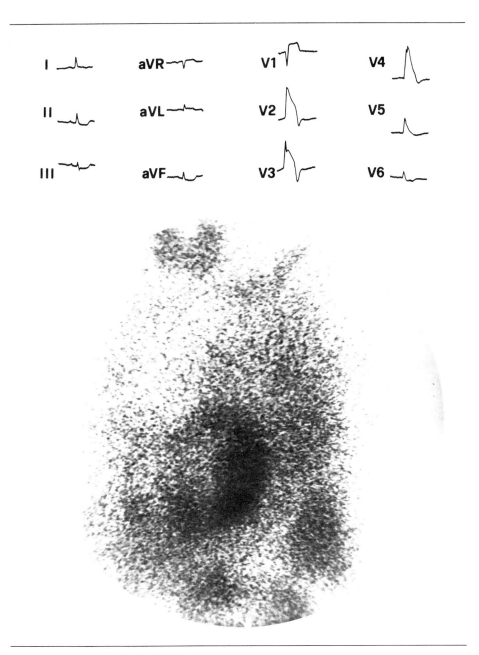

Figure 4-2 Marked reduction in ^{201}Tl activity is found in the anteroseptal wall of the left ventricle during spontaneous ST segment elevation at rest (ECG leads V1–V5).

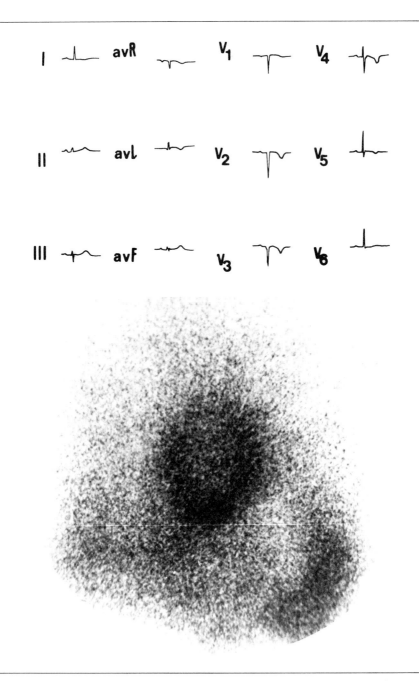

Figure 4-3 Pathological Q waves in leads V1–V3 in the basal state, attributable to old myocardial infarction and accompanied by normal myocardial distribution of ^{201}Tl .

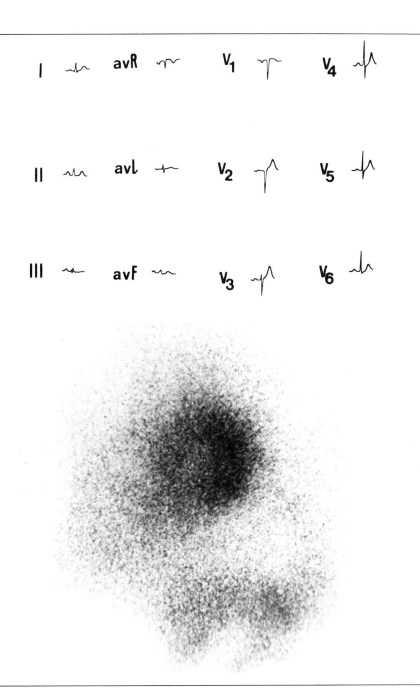

Figure 4-4 Transient normalization of T waves in the precordial leads with typical anginal pain and associated with an extensive perfusion defect involving the anteroseptal and adjacent inferior left ventricular walls.

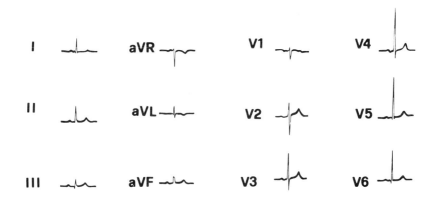

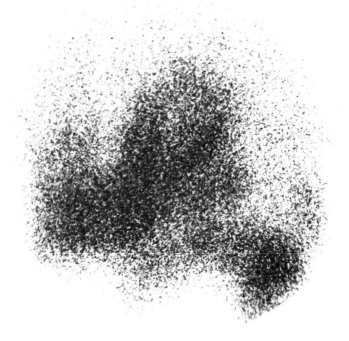

Figure 4-5 Normal ECG and ^{201}Tl scintigram (left anterior oblique projection) recorded in the basal state.

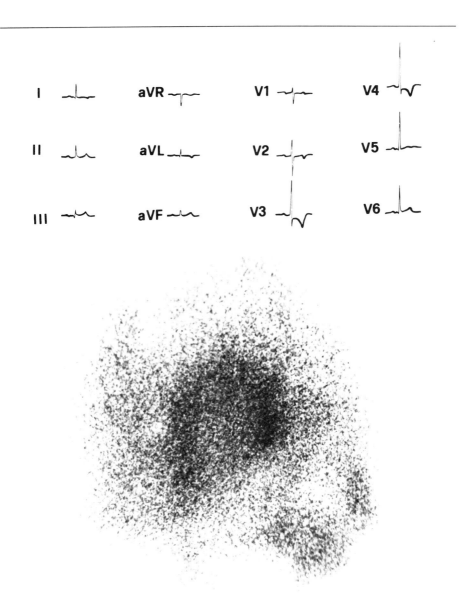

Figure 4-6 Scintigram shows a large, diffuse defect in the anteroseptal and inferior left ventricular walls during angina, with ST segment depression and inversion of T waves in leads V2-V4.

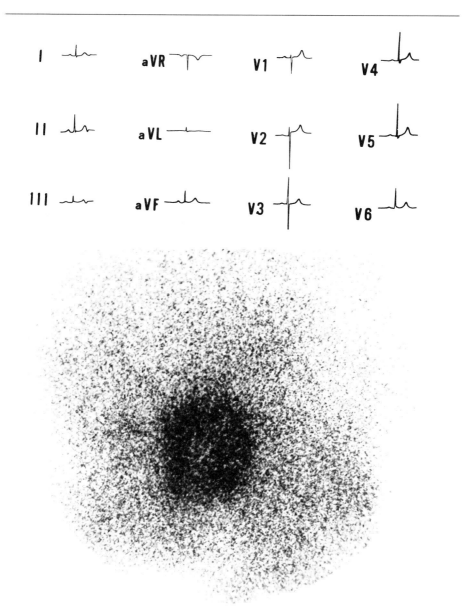

Figure 4-7 Basal ECG and ^{201}Tl scintigram in a patient with effort-induced angina.

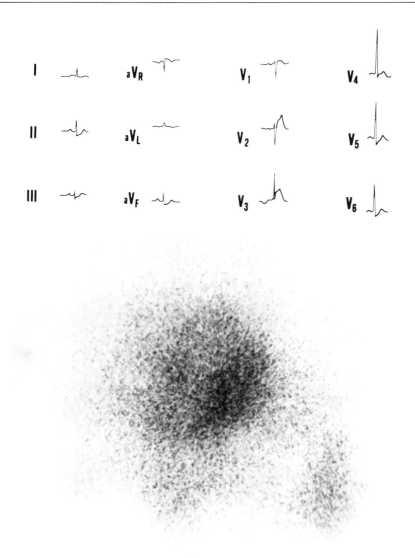

Figure 4-8 Effort-induced ST segment elevation in leads V1–V3, accompanied by a massive perfusion defect in the anteroseptal and inferior walls. ECG leads II, III, and aVF show ST segment depression.

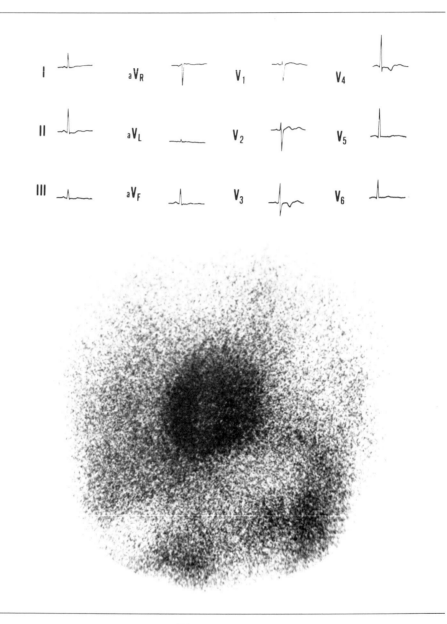

Figure 4-9   Resting basal ECG and ^{201}Tl scintigram.

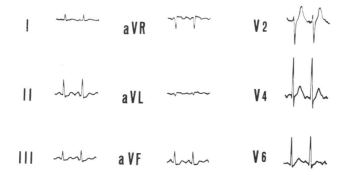

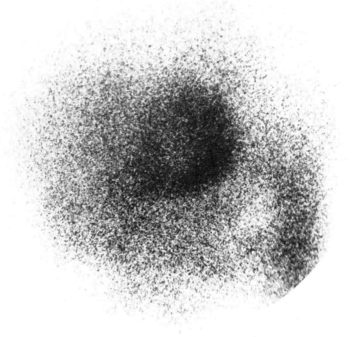

Figure 4-10 Reduction of ^{201}Tl activity in the anteroseptal wall of the left ventricle during effort-induced normalization of T waves in the precordial ECG leads.

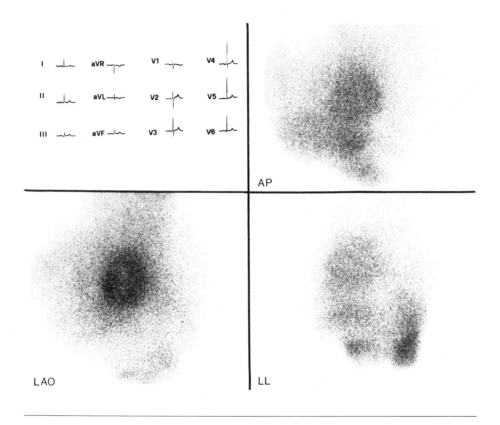

Figure 4-11   ECG and anterior, left anterior oblique, and left lateral scintigrams in the basal state.

References

Biagini, A.; Rovai, D.; Maseri, A., et al. 1978. Comparison of the double product determined during angina at rest and during atrial pacing: Diagnostic significance. In *Transactions of the European Society of Cardiology*, Brighton (England), 1978, vol. 1, 194.

Chierchia, S.; Brunelli, C.; Simonetti, I. et al. 1980. Sequence of events in angina at rest: Primary reduction in coronary flow. *Circulation* 61:759–68.

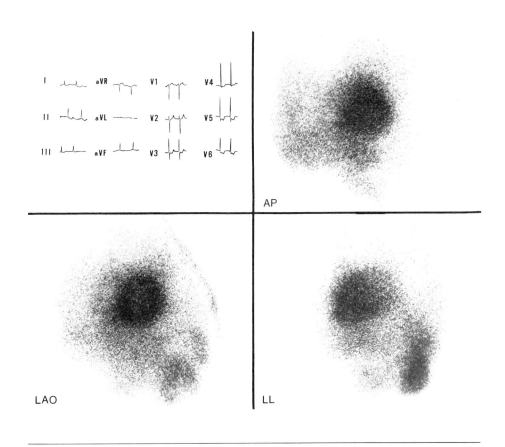

Figure 4-12 No defect of ^{201}Tl activity is seen in spite of unequivocal ischemic
ST segment changes induced by effort.

Curry, R. C.; Pepine, C. J.; Sabom, M. D., et al. 1977. Effects of ergono-
vine in patients with or without coronary artery disease. *Circulation*
56:803–09.

Dhurandhar, R. W.; Watt, D. L.; Silver, M. D., et al. 1972. Prinzmetal's
variant form of angina with arteriographic evidence of coronary arterial
spasm. *Am. J. Cardiol.* 30:902–05.

L'Abbate, A.; Biagini, A.; Michelassi, G., et al. 1979. Myocardial kinetics of thallium and potassium in man. *Circulation* 60:776–85.

Love, W. D.; Ishihara, Y.; Lyon, L. D., et al. 1968. Differences in the relationship between coronary blood flow and myocardial clearance of isotopes of potassium, rubidium and cesium. *Am. Heart J.* 76:353–55.

Marzilli, M.; L'Abbate, A.; Ballestra, A. M., et al. 1977. Coronary arteriographic findings during spontaneous angina with S-T segment depression. Abstract 312, *Circulation*, Part II, vol. 56, no. 4, pp. III-83, October 1977.

Maseri, A.; Mimmo, R.; Chierchia, S., et al. 1975. Coronary spasm as a cause of acute myocardial ischemia in man. *Chest* 68:625–33.

Maseri, A.; Parodi, O.; Severi, S., et al. 1976. Transient reduction of myocardial blood flow, demonstrated by thallium-201 scintigraphy, as a cause of variant angina. *Circulation* 54:280–88.

Maseri, A.; Pesola, A.; Marzilli, M., et al. 1977. Coronary vasospasm in angina pectoris. *Lancet* 2:713–17.

Maseri, A.; Severi, S.; Chierchia, S., et al. 1978. Characteristics, incidence and pathogenetic mechanism of "primary" angina at rest. In *Primary and secondary angina pectoris*, edited by A. Maseri, G. A. Klassen, and M. Lesch, 265-72. New York: Grune & Stratton.

Maseri, A.; Severi, S.; De Nes, M., et al. 1978. "Variant" angina: One aspect of a continuous spectrum of vasospastic myocardial ischemia. Pathogenetic mechanisms, estimated incidence, clinical and coronary arteriographic findings in 138 patients. *Am. J. Cardiol.* 42:1019–35.

Moir, T. W.; and Debra, D. W. 1967. Effect of left ventricular hypertension, ischemic and vasoactive drugs on the myocardial distribution of coronary flow. *Circ. Res.* 21:65–74.

Mudge, G.; Grossman, W.; Mills, R. M., et al. 1976. Reflex increase in coronary vascular resistance in patients with ischemic heart disease. *N. Engl. J. Med.* 295:1333–37.

Oliva, P. V.; Potts, D. E.; and Pluss, R. G. 1973. Coronary arterial spasm in Prinzmetal angina: Documentation by coronary arteriography. *N. Engl. J. Med.* 288:745–51.

Parodi, O.; Uthurralt, N.; Severi, S., et al. 1981. Transient reduction of regional myocardial perfusion during angina at rest with S-T segment depression or normalization of negative T waves. *Circulation* 63:1238–47.

Prinzmetal, M.; Ekemecki, A.; Kennamer, R., et al. 1960. Variant form of angina pectoris: Previously undelineated syndrome. *J.A.M.A.* 174:1794–1800.

Prinzmetal, M.; Kennamer, R.; Merliss, R., et al. 1959. Angina pectoris: I. A variant form of angina pectoris. Preliminary report. *Am. J. Med.* 27:375–88.

Specchia, G.; Severi, S.; Falcone, C., et al. 1979. Coronary arterial spasm as a cause of exercise-induced S-T segment elevation in patients with variant angina. *Circulation* 59:948–54.

Yasue, H.; Omote, S.; Takizawa, A., et al. 1979. Circadian varieties of exercise capacity in patients with Prinzmetal's variant angina: Role of exercise-induced coronary arterial spasm. *Circulation* 59:938–48.

5 Stable Angina

John E. Morch, M.D.

Department of Nuclear Medicine
Royal Jubilee Hospital
Victoria, British Columbia, Canada

The illustrations in this chapter were prepared by the Department of Nuclear Medicine, Royal Jubilee Hospital, Vancouver, British Columbia.

The distribution of thallium-201 (^{201}Tl) is proportional to myocardial blood flow (Strauss, Harrison, et al., 1975; Nishiyama, Adolph, et al., 1982). However, the specific effect of coronary artery narrowing on blood flow varies with the animal model and from patient to patient, depending upon the methodology used. In experimental animals, resting blood flow is normal with coronary lumen narrowing of up to 85% (Gould and Lipscomb, 1974; Gould, Wescott, et al., 1978). However, using radioisotope techniques, clinicians can demonstrate regional myocardial blood flow reduction in patients at rest, with coronary artery narrowing of 70% to 80% or more (Cannon, Sciacca, et al., 1975). Although ^{201}Tl is initially distributed proportional to myocardial blood flow, the uptake obtained with luminal narrowing of this range and in patients at rest is often normal (Figures 5-1–5-5).

Recent reports on resting patients with severe coronary artery narrowing, 90% or greater with reduced blood flow, have shown that the uptake of ^{201}Tl is equivalent to normally perfused areas over minutes to hours (Gewirtz, Beller, et al., 1979), with serial images over two to four hours showing a filling-in of any initial defect.

During exercise, however, myocardium supplied by vessels with 70% to 80% or greater luminal narrowing will have relatively less flow than the myocardium supplied by normal vessels with a two- to threefold increase in flow. Distribution of intravenous ^{201}Tl will consequently be greater in the normally perfused areas, and the underperfused or ischemic areas will appear as defects. A defect in an exercise image can only be attributed to ischemia only if it is not seen in the delayed serial or rest studies. Defects caused by myocardial infarction are also seen in exercise images but, in contrast, persist in the delayed serial and rest studies. (For further discussion of the theoretical basis for thallium imaging, see Chapter 4.)

NORMAL PLANAR ^{201}Tl IMAGES

In the normal myocardium, ^{201}Tl is distributed to show uniform uptake in all views (Figure 5-1). The anterior (Ant), left anterior oblique (LAO), and left lateral (LL) projections are commonly used for analysis and are divided into the segments shown in Figure 5-2. There is overlap of coronary artery distribution as shown on the images of most projections. The LAO view has minimal overlap and permits distinction among the circumflex, left anterior descending, and posterior interventricular branches (Ritchie, Hamilton, et al., 1978). Not all segments are seen in the LL projection.

Two factors affect the appearance of images in the various projections. First, the mass of myocardium facing the gamma camera at right angles to the crystal surface is an important influence. In some projections the mass of myocardium is seen "end on" and shows increased activity. In other areas the mass and, consequently, activity are less when the myocardial wall is "face on" or parallel to the crystal surfaces. Second, there

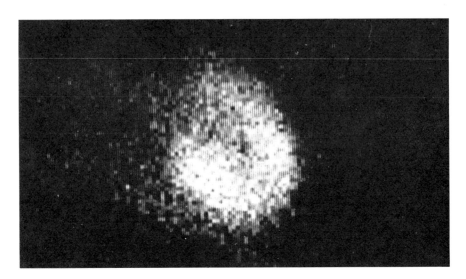

(a) Anterior view

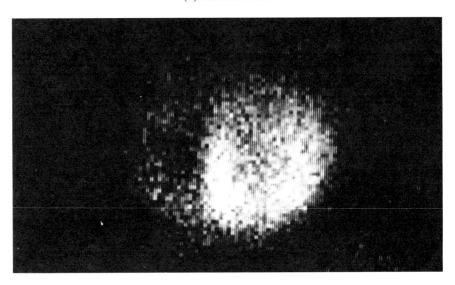

(b) Left anterior oblique view

Figure 5-1 Normal thallium image.

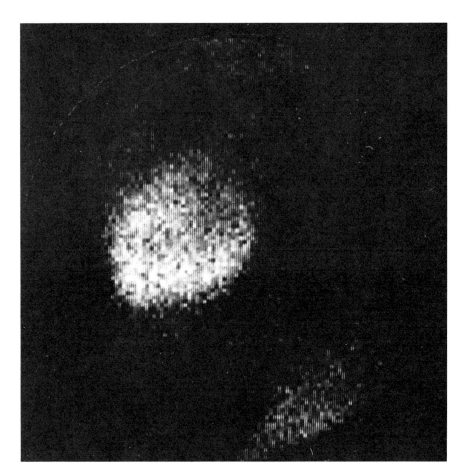

(c) Lateral view

Figure 5-1 (Continued)

are differences in the distance of various parts of the myocardium to the crystal surface—for example, the posterior wall in the Ant and LAO projections. Therefore, the myocardial images appear to be horseshoe or oval in shape, with the ventricular cavity in the center lacking in activity (Figure 5-1). Some variation in overall appearance of the images may occur in specific projections. For example, in the LAO projection, the majority of patients present a doughnut image; however, in some patients a horseshoe shape is seen because of the superiorly situated aortic opening in the LAO view, because of the mitral valve opening.

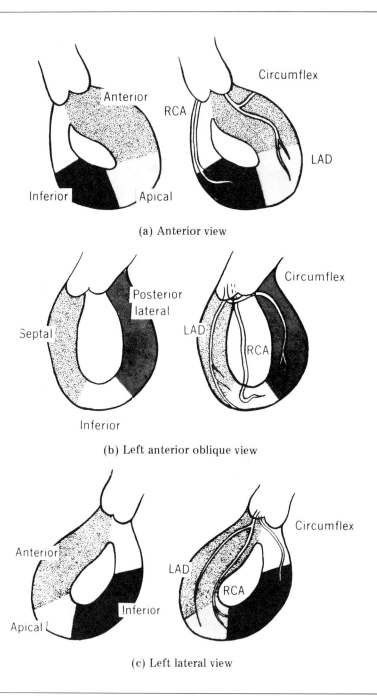

(a) Anterior view

(b) Left anterior oblique view

(c) Left lateral view

Figure 5-2 Nomenclature of segments and coronary artery anatomy.

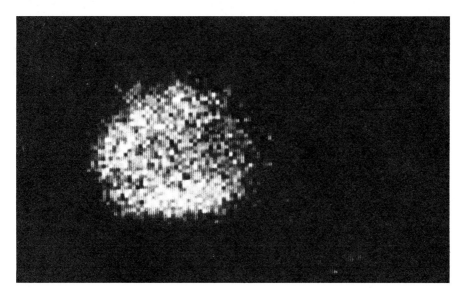

Lateral

Figure 5-3 Normal apical thinning.

Specific areas may have decreased activity as part of a normal variation, for example, the apex in the LAO projection (Figure 5-3) when less mass or thinning is evident. Similarly, normals may have decreased activity in the posterior area in the Ant projection (Figure 5-4) or superior part of the lateral aspect in the LAO projection (Figure 5-5).

Imaging following exercise generally produces better images because of improved myocardium-to-background ratios—that is, an increase in myocardial uptake relative to the structures around the heart. Imaging done two to four hours after isotope administration, called the "wash-in" or redistribution image, is used commonly as a substitute for rest imaging.

TECHNIQUE FOR REST AND EXERCISE ^{201}Tl IMAGING

Rest Imaging

The resting patient is given an intravenous injection of 1.5 to 2.0 mCi of ^{201}Tl in the standing position, to reduce uptake by the splanchnic viscera and lungs. After one to two minutes, imaging in the various projections is started with a convenient display format. If a defect is demonstrated, serial images at two to four hours after the initial study are needed to distinguish infarction from ischemia.

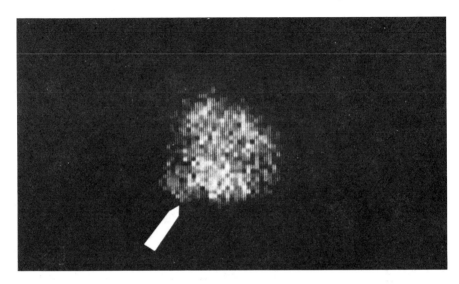

Immediate anterior

Figure 5-4 Normal decrease in thallium uptake in posterior portion of inferior segment in the anterior view.

Exercise Imaging

The fasting patient is exercised on a treadmill or bicycle ergometer, with an intravenous line in place and appropriate ECG monitoring to detect ST-T changes and arrhythmias occurring during the test. Blood pressure is measured regularly by sphygmomanometer, and a defibrillator should be on stand-by. To obtain optimal diagnostic images, exercise is carried out according to the Bruce protocol or similar graded routines until the patient achieves target heart rate or develops angina symptoms. Indications for termination of the test are ST segment depression, arrhythmias, and/or hypotension. Thallium-201, 1.5 to 2.0 mCi, is injected intravenously, and if possible the patient continues at the same level, or a reduced level if symptomatic, for 30 to 90 seconds. Imaging is then carried out as promptly as possible as described for the rest study.

INTERPRETATION OF PLANAR ^{201}Tl IMAGES

The segments of the planar images, whether in analog or digital form, are analyzed visually for uniformity and for the amount of ^{201}Tl uptake, and then compared to other segments. Uptake in a specific segment is compared to that in adjacent segments in the same projection. If decreased uptake is suggested in a segment, it is checked in other projections for confirmation. A marked thinning of a segment may also indicate decreased

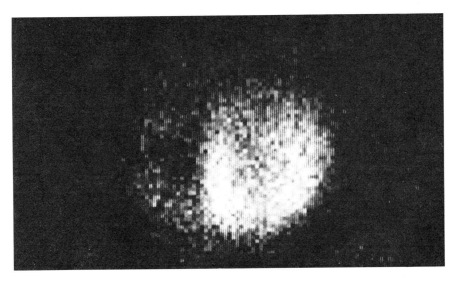

LAO

Figure 5-5 Normal decrease in superior portion of septal segment in left anterior oblique view.

uptake. If the defect persists in a delayed serial image or a rest study, infarction is likely. If the defect disappears on delayed serial rest imaging, then ischemia is the most probable cause. Where two independent observers analyze the images, it is helpful to score the segments: normal uptake, 0; equivocal defect, 1+; and positive defect, 2+. An average score for any segment of 1+ or greater constitutes a defect. Optimally, a defect should be seen in a specific segment in more than one projection, but a 2+ defect in even one projection is generally considered adequate. Because some segments are less clearly visualized or not seen at all in certain projections, it is unreasonable to require that the defect be seen in all three possible views. Any segment with a defect must be compared with a rest or redistribution image of the same segment to decide whether ischemia or scarring has been demonstrated. When possible, interpretation by more than one observer with averaging of scores will increase sensitivity and specificity.

Recognition of the particular coronary artery involved is highly specific in certain segments, such as the anterior wall and septum for the left anterior descending artery, inferior wall for the right coronary artery, and proximal lateral wall for the left circumflex coronary artery. However, left circumflex coronary artery sensitivity is lower than right coronary or left anterior descending artery. There is reduced sensitivity for identifying specifically narrowed vessels in triple vessel disease, where it appears that only the most ischemic segment may be seen (Rigo, Bailey, et al., 1980). Improved sensitivity without loss of specificity was reported by Maddahi, Garcia, et al. (1981), using computer techniques.

Although most analyses are performed by visual methods, the computer is being increasingly used to obtain objective diagnostic data. Most methods utilize a background subtraction technique with comparison of activity in specific regions to normal values. One study (Berger, Watson, et al., 1979) found that the computer demonstrated images critical to the diagnosis in 20% of patients. Maddahi, Garcia, et al. (1981) showed improved sensitivity and specificity using circumferential profiles of thallium distribution compared to visual analysis. Continued reports of refinements in computer analysis can be expected.

REDISTRIBUTION STUDIES OR "WASH-IN" IMAGING

Redistribution studies can be used as a substitute for rest imaging. The mechanism by which a defect seen on exercise or at rest is filled in at two to four hours is believed to be a redistribution of ^{201}Tl , not necessarily related to coronary blood flow (Gerry, Becker, et al., 1980). Redistribution is likely because of a differential clearance of ^{201}Tl from the normal compared with the ischemic tissue and an absolute increase in activity in the ischemic area (Nishiyama, Adolph, et al., 1982).

Generally, imaging is performed at one, two, and four hours after the initial study by collecting a predetermined number of counts. Computer manipulation of the data, including background subtraction and normalization of counts to levels seen in the initial study, has improved the quality and reliability of "wash-in" imaging. If a defect seen on exercise disappears in the wash-in image, it can be assumed that the initial defect was a result of ischemia (Figures 5-6a, 5-6b, 5-7a, and 5-7b). If fill-in does not occur, new or old infarction is the most likely diagnosis (Figure 5-8).

Confusion in the interpretation of wash-in images may arise if uptake is poor, if partial fill-in occurs, or if new defects resulting from reverse distribution are seen in areas previously normally perfused. The mechanism of reverse redistribution is not understood, but it may be another indicator of coronary artery disease (Hecht, Hopkins, et al., 1979). Berger, Watson, et al. (1981) reported a refinement in the analysis of washout images by constructing time-activity curves from selected regions of interest in serial washout images. The value of establishing the washout rate was not confirmed by Becker, Rogers, et al. (1980).

CLINICAL APPLICATIONS OF ^{201}Tl IMAGING

The usefulness of imaging is improved in patients with stable angina if final interpretation is made in the light of other clinical information, such as symptoms, rest, and the stress ECG. However, to better appreciate the

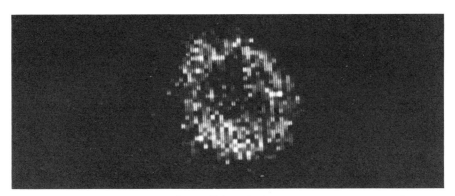

Immediate anterior

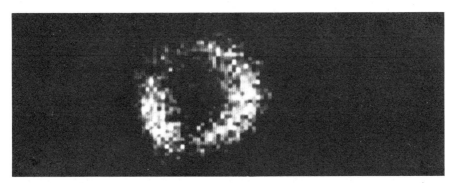

Immediate 45° LAO

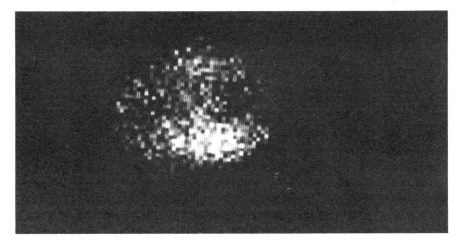

Immediate lateral

Figure 5-6a Septal, apical, and anterior segment defects.

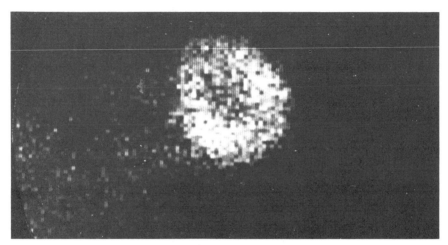

Delayed anterior

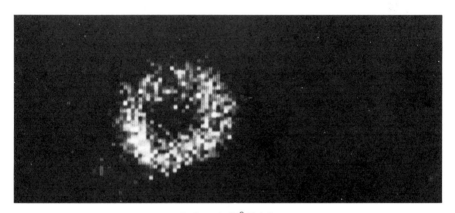

Delayed 45° LAO

Figure 5-6b Delayed (4-hour) image with improved perfusion in previous defects. Some reduction of apical uptake persists.

applications of the technique, its sensitivity and specificity should be known. A number of reports indicate that sensitivity ranges from 71% to 85% (Bodenheimer, Banka, et al., 1980) and specificity from 79% to 92%. When stress ECG results are considered in conjunction with ^{201}Tl imaging, sensitivity is improved by 3% to 15% (Bodenheimer, Banka, et al., 1980). Using quantitative analysis on serial imaging, Berger, Watson, et al. (1981) reported 91% sensitivity, 90% specificity, and 97% predictive accuracy.

The most common use of myocardial imaging (Table 5-1) is in the diagnosis of patients with ischemic-like pain in the chest who have a nega-

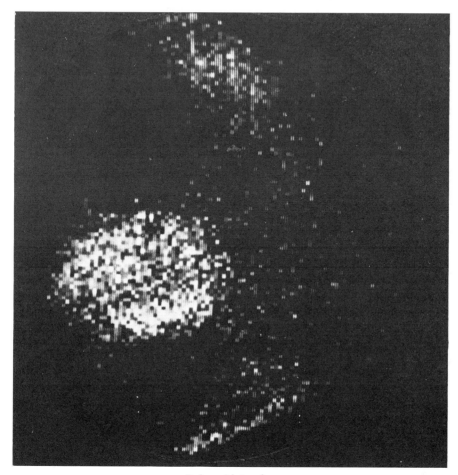

Delayed lateral

Figure 5-6b (Continued)

Table 5-1 Clinical uses for ^{201}Tl Imaging

Ischemic-type chest pain but nondiagnostic stress ECG

Atypical chest pain with positive stress ECG

Atypical chest pain with negative stress ECG

Asymptomatic with positive stress ECG

Evaluation of scarred vs. normal myocardium

Follow-up of patients with progression of disease after selective
coronary arteriograms or aortocoronary bypass

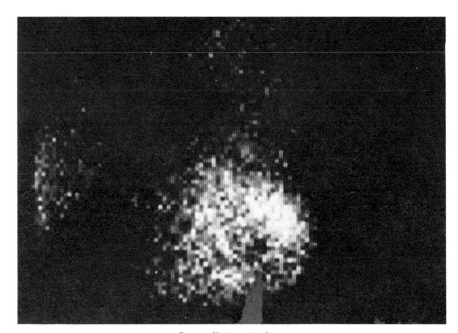

Immediate anterior

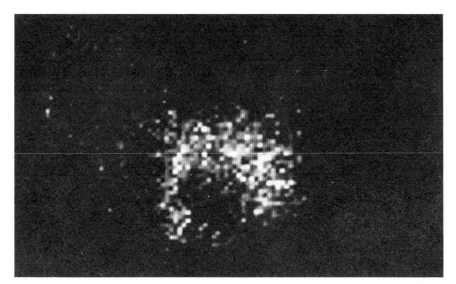

Immediate 45° LAO

Figure 5-7a Inferior and septal defect in uptake.

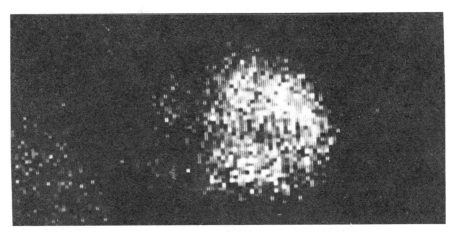

Delayed anterior

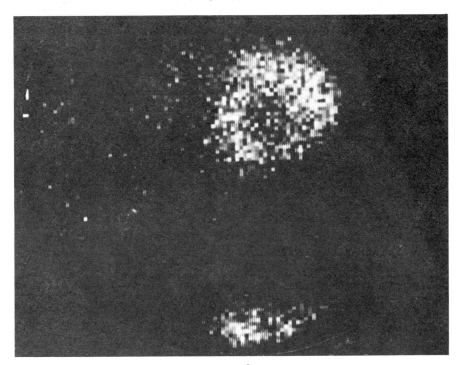

Delayed 45° LAO

Figure 5-7b Delayed (4-hour) image with improved uptake in all segments.

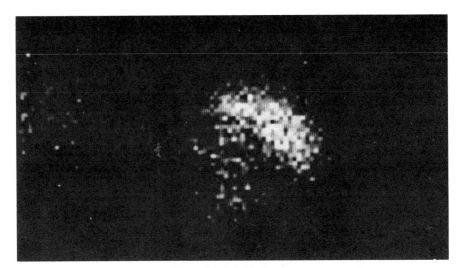

Immediate anterior

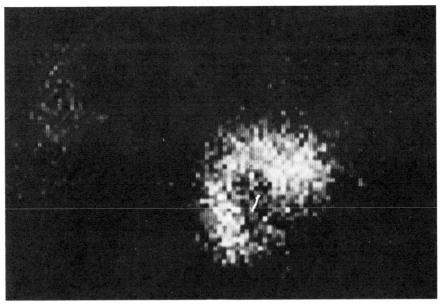

LAO

Figure 5-8 Defect in thallium uptake in inferior segment. No change was seen on 4-hour delayed image indicating infarction.

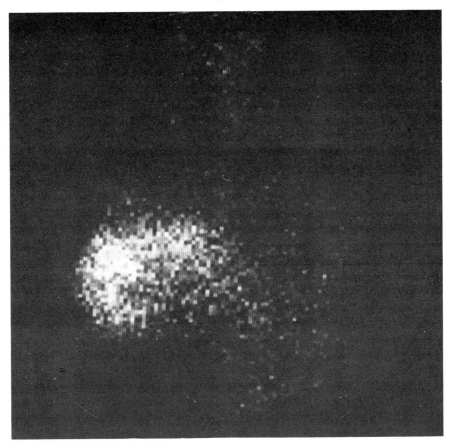

Immediate lateral

Figure 5-8 (Continued)

tive or noninterpretable stress ECG (noninterpretable because of inability to reach the target heart rate or because of conduction abnormalities of left ventricular hypertrophy). McCarthy, Blood, et al. (1979) showed perfusion defects in 81% of 32 patients with nondiagnostic ECGs.

Thallium-201 imaging is also used to determine the localization and extent of myocardial ischemia resulting from exercise. Similarly, localization and size of a myocardial infarct can be determined from the rest image, and this information is very useful for patient management and prognosis.

Follow-up studies are also helpful in the determination of progression in coronary artery disease, especially if the patient has had selective coronary arteriograms or bypass surgery. Several reports have described improved perfusion on repeat postoperative testing (Ritchie, Narahara, et al., 1977; Greenberg, Hart, et al., 1978). If patients deteriorate, myocardial imaging could be helpful in determining noninvasively whether the graft has occluded or there is progression of distal disease in the non-grafted vessels.

Thallium-201 imaging can also be of value in the diagnosis of patients with asymptomatic positive ECG stress tests as detected through routine screening. However, general screening for coronary artery disease is not at present very productive, because of its less than ideal sensitivity, except in selected populations with a high incidence of disease (Ritchie, Hamilton, et al., 1978). Imaging patients with an expected prevalence of disease in the 30% to 70% range should be the most productive.

Limitations

False positives or defects in patients with normal coronary arteries are referred to elsewhere. Image defects in association with normal coronary arteries have been reported in patients with other clinically recognizable cardiac lesions, such as muscular subaortic stenosis (Huckell, Staniloff, et al., 1978), mitral valve prolapse (Staniloff, Huckell, et al., 1978), and cardiomyopathies (Huckell, Staniloff, et al., 1977). Other authors have not reported defects with mitral valve prolapse (Gaffney, Wohl, et al., 1978; Massie, Botvinick, et al., 1978), and differences in the patient population studied (for example, the severity of exercise-induced chest pain) may explain the discrepancies. At this time, diagnosis of defects in patients with other cardiac lesions must be made with caution.

PLANAR ^{201}Tl IMAGING FOLLOWING PHARMACOLOGIC VASODILATION

Gould described a promising technique utilizing the coronary vasodilation properties of intravenous dipyridamole (Albro, Gould, et al., 1978; Gould, Wescott, et al., 1978). Lepp, Boucher, et al. (1982) reported a sensitivity of 93% and specificity of 80%. The drug is infused at 0.145 mg/kg/min for three to four minutes or less if symptoms develop. Thallium-201 is then injected with the patient in an upright position. If symptoms of chest pain or ST segment depression develop, the infusion is stopped. When these symptoms persist, 100 mg of aminophylline can be given intravenously, with almost immediate relief.

Excellent myocardial uptake can usually be demonstrated without exercising the patient and early reports suggest improved sensitivity and specificity (Albro, Gould, et al., 1978). In our experience, good images can be obtained with lower doses of ^{201}Tl, such as 1.25 mCi, resulting in considerable reduction in cost. This technique can also be useful in patients unable to reach target heart rates or unable to exercise because of peripheral vascular disease, musculoskeletal disorders, or a postsurgery condition. In our comparison of pre- and postoperative imaging using dipyridamole, a 95% predictive accuracy was achieved for graft patency where a preoperative defect was shown (Murphy, Bonet, et al., 1979). There are obvious limitations with multiple grafts to vessels with perfusion areas in close proximity, for example, in the case of the diagonal and left anterior descending arteries. In addition, patients in whom a preoperative defect cannot be demonstrated will not benefit from this technique for the determination of graft patency.

COLD PRESSOR ^{201}Tl SCINTIGRAPHY

As an alternative to pharmacological vasodilatation in patients unable to exercise adequately, a cold pressure test has been advocated (Ahmad, Dubiel, et al., 1982). The usual dose of ^{201}Tl was inserted after 30 seconds of cold pressor stimulation. The sensitivity in detecting coronary artery disease was 40% in patients with seven-vessel disease, 91% in patients with two-vessel disease, and 100% in patients with three-vessel disease. This technique may be useful in selected patients.

TOMOGRAPHIC IMAGING IN STABLE ANGINA

Many of the limitations of planar imaging, such as those resulting from superimposition of the anterior and posterior walls of the heart, can be avoided by tomographic techniques using either positron-emitting or gamma-emitting isotopes. Because positron-emitting methods are expensive and limited to centers with access to a cyclotron, they will not be discussed. The technique for using gamma-emitting isotopes is described in Chapter 1. Basically, through the use of a computer and a special rotating slant-hole or multiple-hole collimator, or rotating camera, a three-dimensional reconstruction of an image is possible. Transverse "slicing" along the long axis of the heart, or "bread loafing," permits in-depth visualization of the myocardium (Figure 5-9). Transmural distribution of isotope perfusion can be delineated circumferentially in any segment.

Our preliminary studies suggest that tomographic imaging with the pinhole collimator may be more specific and sensitive than planar methods. An increase in specificity and sensitivity has been reported by Vogel, Kirch, et al. (1979) and others. Vogel, Alderson, et al. (1980), using a quantitative circumferential profile interpretation of the tomograms, reported a specificity of 96% and a sensitivity of 86%.

Single photon emission tomography (SPECT) for ^{201}Tl has been performed with the rotating gamma camera and has been compared to seven-pinhole tomography and planar imaging (Tamaki, Mukai, et al., 1981). Although seven-pinhole tomography achieved better results than

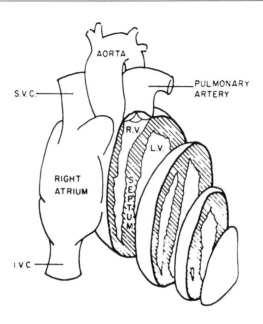

Figure 5-9 Tomographic display of thallium image (after Vogel, R.A.; Kirch, D. L.; LeFree, M. T., et al., 1979 *Am. J. Cardiol.* 43:787–93).

did planar imaging, the SPECT results were best, with a 96% sensitivity and 89% specificity. However, the SPECT equipment is significantly more expensive and complex to use.

Tomographic Imaging Following Pharmacologic Vasodilation

A further extension of this technique has been described by Francisco, Go, et al. (1979) using dipyridamole; they report 92% sensitivity and 95% specificity, with a 95% positive and 91% negative predictive value. Our data support this view, and limited comparisons of exercise and dipyridamole coronary vasodilatation imaging suggest that comparable results can be obtained. However, larger numbers of patients will have to be studied in order to establish the value of this method.

COMPARISON OF ^{201}Tl MYOCARDIAL IMAGING AND EXERCISE RADIONUCLEAR ANGIOGRAPHY IN CORONARY ARTERY DISEASE

Thallium-201 myocardial imaging and exercise radionuclear angiography measure different parameters of cardiac function. Thallium-201 imaging measures myocardial perfusion and radionuclear angiography measures ejection fraction (global and regional) and wall motion. However, both have good specificity and sensitivity for the diagnosis of coronary artery disease. Which test should be used? The decision is determined on clinical grounds. For radionuclear angiography, the patient must be in sinus rhythm and be able to pedal a bicycle in the supine position. Alternatively, for ^{201}Tl imaging, the patient is required to walk on a treadmill or receive intravenous vasodilators. Some reports indicate that the ejection fraction shows a wide variety of response and is an insensitive marker of coronary artery disease. Other studies (Caldwell, Hamilton, et al., 1980) suggest that an abnormal exercise ejection fraction was more sensitive than a new thallium abnormality (93% vs. 71%). However, the addition of computer analysis of thallium imaging probably results in comparable sensitivity.

In summary, the two techniques measure different parameters but both have impressive sensitivity and specificity for the detection of coronary artery disease. The choice will be determined on clinical grounds and the nature of the information required. If both are performed, all patients with coronary artery disease can be detected (Caldwell, Hamilton, et al., 1980).

References

Ahmad, M.; Dubiel, J. P.; and Haibach, H. 1982. Cold pressor thallium-201 myocardial scintigraphy in the diagnosis of coronary artery disease. *Am. J. Cardiol.* 50:1253.

Albro, P. C.; Gould, L. K.; Westcott, J. R., et al. 1978. Noninvasive assessment of coronary stenoses by myocardial imaging during pharmacologic vasodilation. *Am. J. Cardiol.* 42:751-60.

Becker, L. C.; Rogers, W. J.; and Edwards, A. C. 1980. Limitations of thallium "washout rate" measurements after exercise for detection of coronary artery stenoses. Abstract, *Circulation* 62 (suppl. II):III-231.

Berger, B. C.; Watson, D. D.; Taylor, G. J., et al. 1981. Quantitative thallium-201 exercise scintigraphy for detection of coronary artery disease. *J. Nucl. Med.* 22:585-93.

Bodenheimer, M. W.; Banka, V. S.; and Helfant, R. H. 1980. Nuclear cardiology. II. The role of myocardial perfusion imaging using thallium-201 in the diagnosis of coronary heart disease. *Am. J. Cardiol.* 45:674-84.

Caldwell, J. H.; Hamilton, G. W.; Sorensen, S. G., et al. 1980. The detection of coronary artery disease with radionuclide techniques: A comparison of rest-exercise thallium imaging and ejection fraction response. *Circulation* 61:610-19.

Cannon, P. J.; Sciacca, R. R.; Fowler, D. L., et al. 1975. Measurement of regional myocardial blood flow in man: Description and critique of the method using xenon-133 and a scintillation camera. *Am. J. Cardiol.* 36:783–92.

Francisco, D.; Go, R.; Vankirk, O., et al. 1979. Tomographic thallium-201 perfusion scintigrams following maximal coronary vasodilatation with dipridamole. Abstract, *Circulation* 60 (suppl. II):174.

Gaffney, F. A.; Wohl, A. J.; Blomqvist, G. C., et al. 1978. Thallium-201 myocardial perfusion studies in patients with the mitral valve prolapse syndrome. *Am. J. Med.* 64:21–26.

Gerry, J. L.; Becker, L. C.; Flaherty, J. T., et al. 1980. Evidence for a flow-independent contribution to the phenomenon of thallium redistribution. *Am. J. Cardiol.* 45:58–62.

Gewirtz, H.; Beller, G. A.; Strauss, H. W., et al. 1979. Transient defects of resting thallium scans in patients with coronary artery disease. *Circulation* 59:707–21.

Gould, L. K.; and Lipscomb, K. 1974. Effects of coronary stenoses on coronary flow reserve and resistance. *Am. J. Cardiol.* 34:48–55.

Gould, L. K.; Wescott, J. R.; Albro, P. C., et al. 1978. Noninvasive assessment of coronary stenoses by myocardial imaging during pharmacologic coronary vasodilation. *Am. J. Cardiol.* 40:279–87.

Greenberg, B. H.; Hart, R.; Botvinick, E. H., et al. 1978. Thallium-201 myocardial perfusion scintigraphy to evaluate patients after coronary bypass surgery. *Am. J. Cardiol.* 42:167–76.

Hecht, M. S.; Hopkins, J. M.; Blumfield, D. E., et al. 1979. Reverse redistribution: Worsening of thallium-201 images from exercise to distribution. Abstract, *Circulation* 60 (suppl. II):II-61.

Huckell, V. F.; Staniloff, H. M.; Feiglin, D. H., et al. 1978. The demonstration of segmental perfusion defects in hypertrophic cardiomyopathy imitating coronary artery disease. Abstract, *Am. J. Cardiol.* 41:438.

Huckell, V. F.; Staniloff, H. M.; McLaughlin, P. R., et al. 1977. The implications of segmental perfusion defects in cardiomyopathies using thallium-201. Abstract, *Clin. Res.* 25:227A.

Leppo, J.; Boucher, C. A.; Okada, R. D., et al. 1982. Serial thallium-201 myocardial imaging after dipyridamole infusion: Diagnostic utility in detecting coronary stenoses and relationship to regional wall motion. *Circulation* 66:649–57.

McCarthy, D. M.; Blood, D. K.; Sciacca, R. R., et al. 1979. Single dose myocardial perfusion imaging with thallium-201: Application in patients with non-diagnostic electrocardiographic stress tests. *Am. J. Cardiol.* 43:899–906.

Maddahi, J.; Garcia, E. V.; Berman, D. S., et al. 1981. Improved non-invasive assessment of coronary artery disease by quantitative analysis of regional stress myocardial distribution and washout of thallium-201. *Circulation* 64:924–35.

Massie, B.; Botvinick, E. H.; Shames, D., et al. 1978. Myocardial perfusion scintigraphy in patients with mitral valve prolapse: Its advantages over stress electrocardiography in diagnosing associated coronary artery disease and its implications for the etiology of chest pain. *Circulation* 57:19–26.

Murphy, A.; Bonet, J.; McLaughlin, P., et al. 1979. Noninvasive assessment of early postoperative bypass graft patency. *Circulation* 60:237.

Nishiyama, H.; Adolph, R. J.; Gabel, M., et al. 1982. Effect of coronary blood flow on thallium-201 uptake and washout. *Circulation* 65:534–42.

Okada, R. D.; Boucher, C. A.; Kirshenbaum, H. K., et al. 1980. Improved diagnostic accuracy of thallium-201 stress test using multiple observers and criteria derived from interobserver analysis of variance. *Am. J. Cardiol.* 46:619–24.

Rigo, P.; Bailey, I. K.; Griffith, L. S. C., et al. 1980. Value and limitations of segmental analysis of stress thallium myocardial imaging for localization of coronary artery disease. *Circulation* 61:973–81.

Ritchie, J. L.; Hamilton, G. W.; and Wackers, F. J. T., editors. 1978. *Thallium-201 myocardial imaging*, 57. New York: Raven Press.

Ritchie, J. L.; Narahara, K. A.; Trobaugh, G. B., et al. 1977. Thallium-201 myocardial imaging before and after coronary revascularization. *Circulation* 56:830–36.

Staniloff, H. M.; Huckell, V. F.; Morch, J. E., et al. 1978. Abnormal myocardial perfusion defects in patients with mitral valve prolapse and normal coronary arteries. Abstract, *Am. J. Cardiol.* 41:433.

Strauss, H. W.; Harrison, K.; Langan, J. K., et al. 1975. Thallium-201 for myocardial imaging: Relation of thallium-201 to regional myocardial perfusion. *Circulation* 51:641–45.

Tamaki, N.; Mukai, T.; Ishii, Y., et al. 1981. Clinical evaluation of thallium-201 emission myocardial tomography using a rotating gamma camera: Comparison with seven-pinhole tomography. *J. Nucl. Med.* 22:849–55.

Vogel, R.; Alderson, P.; Berman, D., et al. 1980. A multicenter comparison of standard and seven pinhole tomographic TL-201 scintigraphy. Abstract, *Circulation* 62 (suppl. II):III-9.

Vogel, R. A.; Kirch, D. L.; LeFree, M. T., et al. 1979. Thallium-201 myocardial perfusion scintigraphy: Results of standard multi-pinhole tomographic techniques. *Am. J. Cardiol.* 43:787–93.

Assessment of Myocardial Perfusion by Invasive Techniques: Radiolabeled Particles and Radioactive Diffusible Gases

6

William J. Kostuk, M.D.

Cardiac Investigation Unit
University Hospital
London, Ontario, Canada

This work was supported in part by the Ontario Heart Foundation.

A full assessment of coronary atherosclerotic heart disease includes not only a review of symptoms but also an examination of the coronary anatomy, collateral circulation patterns, and left ventricular function. Selective coronary angiography can define precisely the anatomic site of obstruction in the major coronary arteries, while contrast left ventriculography can assess left ventricular function. Abnormalities in regional wall motion are frequent, and it is of the utmost importance to determine whether these abnormalities are caused by ischemic or scarred myocardium. Such differentiation, although it is often difficult on the basis of angiographic studies alone, is becoming more important with the continuing increase in the numbers of patients being considered for coronary artery bypass surgery (Mundth and Austen, 1975). The delivery of additional blood to an ischemic myocardium can improve myocardial function and relieve ischemic symptoms; however, providing additional blood flow to heavily scarred myocardium is a futile exercise and exposes the patient to needless risk.

Several radionuclide techniques are available to measure myocardial blood flow or perfusion in humans. Myocardial imaging following intravenous injection of thallium-201 or intracoronary injection of radiolabeled particles produces a series of static images that provides a qualitative assessment of blood flow at the moment of injection. On the other hand, the use of radioactive inert gases such as xenon-133 provides a quantitative method for the estimation of myocardial blood flow. This chapter will review both invasive methods.

PERFUSION IMAGING: RADIOLABELED PARTICLES

Myocardial perfusion imaging following the selective intracoronary injection of radiolabeled albumin particles is a direct method for assessing the quality and distribution of the coronary microcirculation (Endo, Yamazaki, et al., 1970; Ashburn, Braunwald, et al., 1971; Weller, Adolph, et al., 1972; Jansen, Judkins, et al., 1973; Hamilton, Ritchie, et al., 1975; Kostuk, 1977). If mixing is adequate, the distribution of these biodegradable particles is proportional to blood flow and reflects the area of myocardial tissue supplied by the coronary artery into which the particles were injected. Perfused myocardium is presumed to be viable while lack of regional perfusion is held to indicate the presence of scar tissue, presumably the result of previous myocardial infarction.

Method of Injection

The use of two radionuclides of differing energy peaks permits one to visualize not only the microcirculation of each coronary artery but also the pattern of collateral circulation. The particles used—macroaggregated albumin—must be of uniform size and proper diameter (20–30 μ) so that they can be trapped in the capillary bed downstream from the injection site. On completion of selective coronary angiography, the catheter tip is removed from the coronary artery and the catheter is flushed with normal saline. In order to avoid contrast-induced hyperemia (Ritchie, Hamilton, et al., 1975) and to permit a return to resting flow, the particles are injected at least two to three minutes after the last injection of contrast material. Following repositioning of the catheter tip in the coronary ostium, the labeled particles are selectively injected into the coronary arteries over one to two seconds. The catheter is then flushed with 3 to 5 mL of normal saline that also contains contrast material, to confirm selective injection. This procedure also permits the operator to determine whether "superselective" injection (circumflex or left anterior descending branches) has occurred owing to streaming of the particles; determining this is particularly important in the presence of a short left main coronary stem.

Technetium-99m (^{99m}Tc) labeled human macroaggregated albumin (MAA) particles are injected into the left coronary artery, while iodine-131 (^{131}I) or indium-113m (^{113m}In) labeled MAA is injected into the right coronary artery. Approximately 20,000 to 30,000 particles of MAA are injected into each coronary artery. Two hundred to three hundred mCi of ^{99m}Tc and 150 mCi of ^{131}I are commonly used. In evaluating the perfusion pattern after aortocoronary venous bypass grafting, the particles may be injected directly into the graft(s). In this situation, ^{131}I labeled particles are injected into the graft(s) and ^{99m}Tc labeled particles into the right and left coronary arteries.

Studies at rest have been performed safely with labeled particles in several thousand patients over the past eight years in different centers (Endo, Yamazaki, et al., 1970; Ashburn, Braunwald, et al., 1971; Weller, Adolph, et al., 1972; Jansen, Judkins, et al., 1973; Hamilton, Ritchie, et al., 1975; Ritchie, Hamilton, et al., 1975; Kostuk, 1977). Experimental work has demonstrated that the number and size of particles used clinically have a wide margin of safety. In animals, over 1.5×10^6 particles were injected before any fall in coronary blood flow could be detected (Weller, Adolph, et al., 1972; Grames, Jansen, et al., 1974).

MYOCARDIAL IMAGING

Technique

Imaging may be delayed for up to three to four hours following injection because the tagged particles are trapped in the coronary capillary circulation for several hours. On completion of cardiac catheterization, the patient is transported to the nuclear medicine department for myocardial imaging with a rectilinear scanner or a scintillation camera. Multiple views are obtained; at a minimum, these views should include the anterior and 45° left anterior oblique positions. The left lateral and right anterior oblique projections may be added if feasible. The use of an imaging device with a dual pulse-height analyzer capability (for ^{131} I and ^{99m} Tc) permits the simultaneous acquisition of the perfusion patterns of the right and left coronary arteries. In addition to permitting separate visualization of the myocardial blood flow of each coronary artery, this technique can provide a "summed" image of overall myocardial perfusion.

Interpretation

Normal myocardial perfusion shows a uniform distribution of the radioactive particles in the injected arterial bed (Figure 6-1). Distribution of the radioactive particles, following injection into the left coronary artery, corresponds to the area perfused by the left anterior descending and circumflex arteries and appears similar to the left ventricular contour as visualized at contrast angiography. Thus, the pattern in the anterior and left lateral projections is ellipsoid, while the pattern in the left anterior oblique projection is reniform or spherical, depending upon the presence or absence of right coronary artery predominance. Following injection into the right coronary artery, the distribution of the radioactive particles shows intense activity inferiorly but little activity anteriorly, and the left anterior oblique view presents a "hockey-stick" pattern. The blade represents perfusion of the inferior wall of the left ventricle while the less dense handle represents blood flow to the right ventricle. When the left coronary artery is dominant, the right coronary image reflects only right ventricular perfusion.

The left anterior oblique projection is most valuable because it provides a distinct separation of the left anterior descending territory anteriorly, the circumflex territory posteriorly, and the right coronary artery distribution inferiorly.

Regions of myocardium supplied by normal coronary arteries, and by coronary arteries with hemodynamically insignificant lesions, show a uniform distribution of the labeled particles. Likewise, in the absence of previous myocardial infarction, regions of myocardium supplied by a coronary artery with a high-grade stenosis or even complete occlusion usually exhibit a normal myocardial particulate image (Figure 6-2). In contrast, myocardial segments that are predominantly composed of scar tissue (the result of previous myocardial infarction) receive little coronary blood flow and thus will show little, if any, particle accumulation. In this instance the abnormal myocardial perfusion image shows a nonuniform pattern of radioactivity with clearly discernible regions of diminished (less than 50% of that expected on the basis of the activity in contiguous areas) or absent activity (Figure 6-3). The dual isotope technique permits the observer to assess the presence or absence of collateral blood flow from one artery to another (Figure 6-2). In a few instances this assessment shows that the collateral perfusion is greater than that expected from the angiographic images.

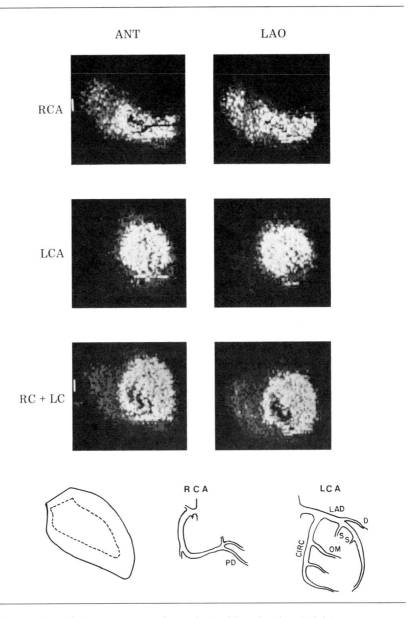

Figure 6-1 Normal perfusion anatomy of a patient with a dominant right coronary artery and no evidence of coronary heart disease. The line diagrams at the bottom represent the normal left ventriculogram (end-diastolic and end-systolic silhouettes in the right anterior oblique view) and the normal coronary artery anatomy. Abbreviations: **RCA**, right coronary artery; **PD**, posterior descending; **LCA**, left coronary artery; **RC + LC**, summation image; **Ant**, anterior; **LAO**, left anterior oblique; **LAD**, left anterior descending; **D**, diagonal branch; **S**, septal perforators; **Circ**, left circumflex; **OM**, obese marginal.

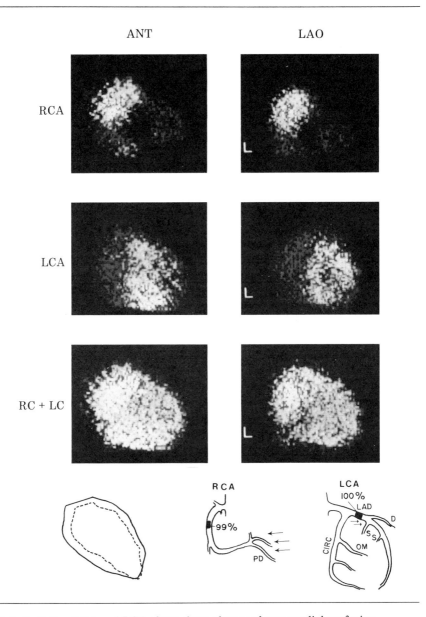

Figure 6-2 Both the RCA and LCA alone show abnormal myocardial perfusion images as a result of proximal coronary artery lesions. The summation image, however, is normal. Note the presence of collateral flow from the RCA to the LAD region and from the LCA to the diaphragmatic segment supplied normally by the RCA. The line diagram indicates the site of disease in the coronary arteries. The arrows indicate the direction of collateral flow. The ventriculogram showed apical akinesis and hypokinesis of the diaphragmatic and anterolateral wall segments. The calculated ejection fraction was 0.47.

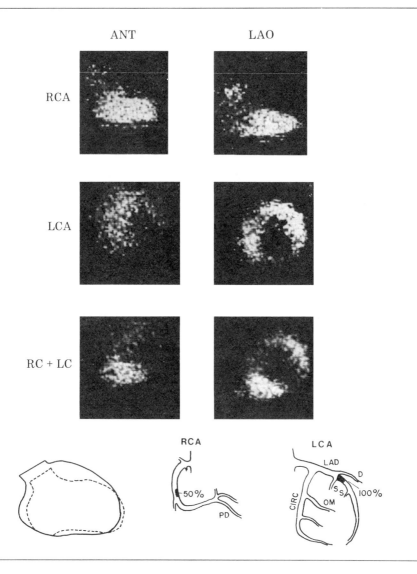

Figure 6-3 Abnormal myocardial perfusion images showing a large perfusion defect involving the anterolateral, apical, and septal segments. The left ventriculograms showed the presence of a left ventricular aneurysm involving the anterolateral and apical segments. The LAD was occluded proximally with mild disease in the RCA. The calculated ejection fraction was 0.36.

Clinical Usefulness and Potential

A normal myocardial perfusion pattern in patients with atypical chest pain and normal coronary arteries provides additional evidence of normality. However, the presence of a myocardial perfusion defect does not invariably indicate the presence of coronary artery disease. Indeed, for meaningful results, the myocardial image must be interpreted together with the angiographic findings. This approach will detect decreased perfusion that has resulted from a superselective injection, i.e., a flow defect caused by a technical abnormality (often the result of an anatomical variation such as a short left main stem coronary artery). Obviously, such a defect is not a true physiologic abnormality. Also, a knowledge of the dominance of the coronary system is essential. Myocardial perfusion abnormalities have been described in patients with cardiomyopathy (Jansen, Judkins, et al., 1973; Kostuk and Chamberlain, 1976a; Bulkley, Rouleau, et al., 1977) as well as valvular heart disease (Kostuk and Chamberlain, 1976a, 1976b; Poe, Eber, et al., 1977) in whom the coronary artery anatomy is angiographically normal. Both of these conditions, in addition to showing cardiomegaly, can show either segmental defects or a diffuse, patchy perfusion pattern (the latter can be the result of too few particles being distributed within a dilated and hypertrophied ventricular chamber). Alternatively, the perfusion defects can represent the patchy and scattered fibrosis that is seen pathologically (Roberts and Ferrans, 1974).

Intracoronary myocardial perfusion studies may be extremely helpful in resolving some of the problems that arise with conventional angiography in patients with coronary atherosclerosis. In these individuals, regardless of the degree of critical stenosis or complete occlusion, if the overall myocardial perfusion images are normal even in the presence of abnormal left ventricular wall motion, the patients have adequate capillary beds and should be good candidates for aortocoronary bypass surgery (Ashburn, Braunwald, et al., 1971; Jansen, Judkins, et al., 1973; Hamilton, Ritchie, et al., 1975; Kostuk, 1977). Conversely, if myocardial perfusion is absent or markedly impaired, it is unlikely that the individual would benefit from a revascularization procedure. In patients with abnormal myocardial perfusion images, the pattern of left ventricular wall motion is invariably abnormal in the area of abnormal myocardial perfusion (Ashburn, Braunwald, et al., 1971; Jansen, Judkins, et al., 1973; Hamilton, Ritchie, et al., 1975; Kostuk, 1977). Hutchins, Bulkley, et al. (1977) showed that the presence of abnormal wall motion on left ventriculography during life was a relatively poor predictor of the presence of ischemic myocardium or myocardial scar at autopsy. The presence of a regional perfusion defect corresponding to a region of abnormal wall motion makes it highly likely that this region represents a transmural scar. Conversely, a normal myocardial perfusion pattern in a region of abnormal wall motion suggests that the myocardial tissue in that region is viable. Thus, intracoronary injection of radiolabeled particles should help in

assessing the significance of abnormal wall motion seen on left ventriculography (Figures 6-2 and 6-4).

Clinically, particulate myocardium perfusion imaging is of value in
predicting myocardial viability in patients undergoing aortocoronary bypass surgery (Hamilton, Murray, et al., 1975; Kirk, Jansen, et al., 1977;
Kostuk and Chamberlain, 1977). Before operation, in one study (Kostuk
and Chamberlain, 1977) of 82 patients undergoing bypass surgery, 67 had
overall normal myocardial perfusion images in spite of the presence of
wall motion abnormalities in 34. After surgery, left ventricular function as
judged by ejection fraction improved in this group: the mean ejection
fraction increased from 56% to 65% (P < 0.01) (Figures 6-2 and 6-4). In
the 15 patients with abnormal myocardial perfusion scans, left ventricular
function improved only if the bypass graft served an area that before operation had normal regional myocardial perfusion. In a larger study of 194
patients undergoing bypass surgery, Kirk, Jansen, et al. (1977) analyzed
the postoperative regional wall motion and the total ventricular function
as expressed by ejection fraction. Of patients with either normal or abnormal left ventricular contraction but normal myocardial perfusion
images before operation, 85% exhibited improvement in their ejection
fraction and over 93% showed a functional improvement in regional wall
movement after operation. Conversely, only 43% of those who had abnormal myocardial perfusion images and abnormal ventriculography before
operation showed any improvement in the postoperative ejection fraction,
while only 24% showed improved regional wall motion (Kirk, Jansen, et
al., 1977).

Gould, Lipscomb, et al. (1974) have proposed that the clinical usefulness of intracoronary particulate injections might be increased by combining the resting myocardial image with one obtained following stress-
induced coronary hyperemia. As noted earlier, in the absence of previous
myocardial infarction, severe disease of the coronary arteries is usually
associated with a normal myocardial particulate scan. Gould and coworkers showed that in atherosclerosis (less than 50% luminal narrowing)
the injection of contrast material may within two minutes alter the distribution of the labeled particles. A stress study such as Gould and coworkers suggested might be of benefit in evaluating the hemodynamic
significance of a questionable angiographically demonstrated coronary
artery lesion. These investigators demonstrated that the intracoronary
injection of contrast media produces such vasodilatation of the coronary
bed that it leads to an immediate four- to fivefold increase in coronary
blood flow (Gould, Lipscomb, et al., 1974). The increase is similar in magnitude to that seen with physiologic stimuli. Thus if the radiolabeled particles are injected into a specific coronary artery during the period of peak
hyperemia (six to ten seconds after the contrast injection), the regions of
myocardium supplied by normal coronary arteries will show no change in
the regional distribution of particles. On the other hand, because of a regional maldistribution of flow, images obtained during hyperemia in myo-

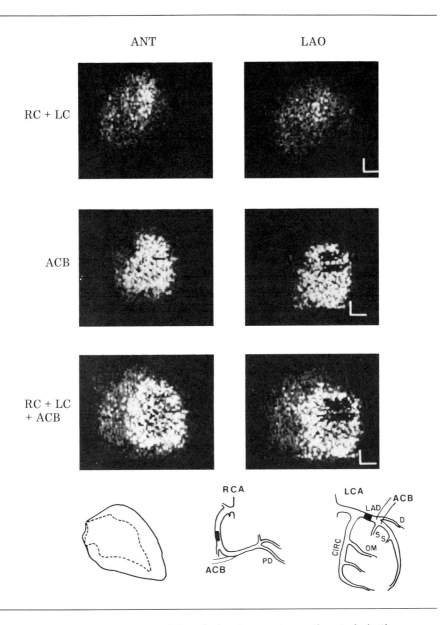

Figure 6-4 Overall normal myocardial perfusion in a postoperative study in the patient shown in Figure 6-3. Most of the myocardial perfusion reaches the muscle through the aortocoronary venous grafts to the LAD and RCA. Note improvement in left ventricular contraction. The calculated ejection fraction was 0.72. **ACB**, aortocoronary bypass grafts.

cardial segments supplied by a significantly diseased coronary artery will have perfusion defects, as compared to the normal rest images.

Limitations

Although the major disadvantage of the labeled particle technique is the absolute dependence upon selective coronary catheterization, a more obvious concern relates to the completeness of particle mixing with the coronary artery blood. Streaming, or superselective injection of the particles, may occur with injection through a single–end-hole coronary catheter and is of particular importance during injection of the left coronary artery. This problem is usually recognized during the contrast study. At the present time it is uncertain whether the information provided by the particulate myocardial perfusion technique is superior to that obtained with myocardial imaging by thallium-201. Thallium-201 is certainly more expensive. Although a single injection can be used to obtain both stress and rest images, the delayed image must be obtained four to six hours after the stress study—making the logistics of obtaining the image somewhat more difficult.

PERFUSION IMAGING: RADIOACTIVE DIFFUSIBLE GAS

Although several different gases have been used to measure myocardial blood flow in man, xenon-133 (^{133}Xe) has been employed most frequently (Cannon, Haft, et al., 1969; Cannon, Dell, et al., 1972a, 1972b; Maseri and Mancini, 1972; Holman, Adams, et al., 1974; Schmidt, Weiss, et al., 1976; Maseri, L'Abbate, et al., 1977). Xenon, a chemically and physiologically inert gas, is lipid-soluble. Following intracoronary injection, it diffuses rapidly into the myocardial cells supplied by the artery—the washout of the gas being a direct function of the capillary blood flow. The radiolabeled technique, on the other hand, does not depend upon the fraction of cardiac output delivered to a vessel. The xenon method, however, requires coronary flow for clearance of the tracer from the myocardium. It is extremely important that more than 95% of an injected bolus be excreted into the expired air during the first passage through the lungs, making both recirculation and background build-up of the tracer a minor problem. Xenon has a physical half-life of 5.3 days and a biologic half-life of one to two minutes.

Method of Injection and Imaging

Following the intracoronary bolus injection of ^{133}Xe (dissolved in 1 to 2 mL of normal saline), an image detector (either a probe or a scintillation camera) is used to record the myocardial washout of the ^{133}Xe that occurs over the next several minutes. This disappearance curve, which is believed to represent myocardial blood flow, is calculated by the Schmidt-Kety method:

$$\frac{F}{W} = \frac{(K)\ (\lambda)}{P}$$

where F/W is the myocardial blood flow per unit weight (mL/100 g/min); K is the rate constant derived from the washout curve; λ is the blood myocardium partition coefficient (which for ^{133}Xe in myocardium is 0.72); and P is the specific gravity of the myocardium (1.05) (Cannon, Weiss, et al., 1977).

The disappearance curve, which is obtained by recording with an external scintillation probe positioned over the precordium, permits the calculation of total or average myocardial blood flow (Horwitz, Curry, et al., 1974). Such determinations are of limited usefulness, since there is considerable overlap between patients with angiographically normal coronary arteries and those with angiographically demonstrated coronary artery disease; in effect, localized regions of reduced flow within the ventricular myocardium are overlooked because of overlap from adjoining normal regions. The net result is an overestimation of average left ventricular flow.

The use of a scintillation camera with a single crystal or multiple crystals permits regional subdivision of the heart. Both Cannon and coworkers (Cannon, Haft, et al., 1969; Cannon, Dell, et al., 1972a) and Maseri and his colleagues (Maseri and Mancini, 1972; Maseri, L'Abbate, et al., 1977) have made impressive advances in the external detection of ^{133}Xe. For four to seven minutes, the scintillation camera records the gamma radiation emitted by the isotope as it diffuses into and out of the myocardial cells (washout) as a function of the myocardial blood flow. Computer processing of the data permits the derivation of the peak counts and the slope of each of the multiple radionuclide washout curves. The use of the Schmidt-Kety formula permits the observer to calculate the myocardial blood flow rates in each of the multiple regions. The pattern of regional myocardial perfusion rates obtained is superimposed upon a tracing of the patient's coronary arteriograms obtained in the same view. Figure 6-5 illustrates myocardial perfusion patterns obtained in different regions of the left ventricle of a normal coronary arteriogram.

Patient Studies

Cannon and his colleagues (Cannon, Haft, et al., 1969; Cannon, Dell, et al., 1972a, b; Dwyer, Dell, et al., 1973; Cannon, Schmidt, et al., 1975; Cannon, Weiss, et al., 1976; Cannon, Weiss, et al., 1977) have evaluated patients with both normal and abnormal coronary arteriograms. In a study of 17 patients with heart disease but normal coronary arteriograms, they found regional variations in the myocardial blood flow rates (Cannon, Weiss, et al., 1977); the average left ventricular flow exceeded right ven-

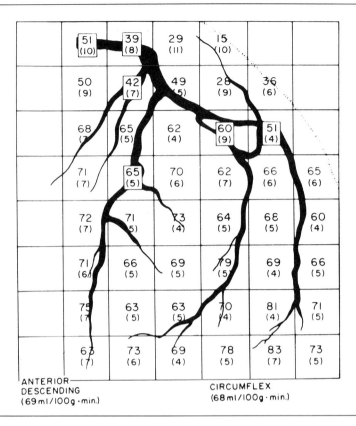

Figure 6-5 The normal myocardial perfusion pattern in a patient with a normal left coronary arteriogram. The computer printout has been aligned and superimposed upon a tracing of the patient's angiogram (LAO projection). (Reproduced, by permission, from Cannon, P. J.; Weiss, M. B.; and Sciacca, R. R. 1977. *Prog. Cardiovasc. Dis.* 20:95–120.)

tricular and right atrial flows. Patients with insignificant coronary stenosis (less than 50% on the coronary arteriogram) and those with isolated left anterior descending coronary artery disease exhibited normal mean myocardial blood flow values at rest (Figure 6-6) (Cannon, Dell, et al., 1972a, b; Dwyer, Dell, et al., 1973; Cannon, Schmidt, et al., 1975; Cannon, Weiss, et al., 1976; Schmidt, Weiss, et al., 1976). Individuals with coronary artery stenosis (greater than 50%) involving two or three major coronary arteries showed a significantly lower mean left ventricular perfusion per given mass of tissue than did control subjects with normal coronary arteriograms. Similarly, patients with localized arterial stenosis of greater than 90%, with or without regions of transmural myocardial infarction, had reduced regional myocardial perfusion at rest (Figure 6-6). Regional myocardial blood flow measurements have been obtained at rest and during

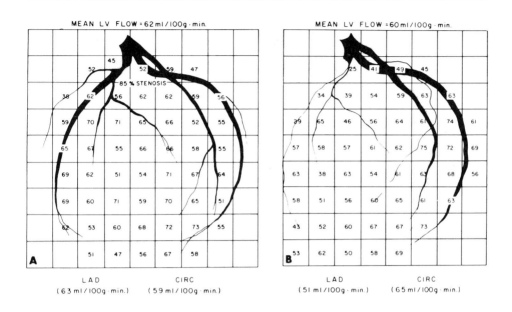

Figure 6-6 (A) The regional myocardial perfusion rates remain normal in this patient despite a significant proximal LAD stenosis. (B) Three months after an anterior myocardial infarction in the same patient, the LAD was completely occluded; the regional myocardial blood flow rates distal to the lesion were significantly lower than elsewhere in the left ventricle. (Reproduced, by permission, from Cannon, P. J.; Weiss, M. B.; and Sciacca, R. R. 1977. *Prog. Cardiovasc. Dis.* 20:95–120.)

atrial pacing in patients with angina pectoris and coronary artery disease (Schmidt, Weiss, et al., 1976; Maseri, L'Abbate, et al., 1977). This type of study assesses the reserve ability of the coronary circulation to increase regional myocardial blood flow. Patients with angiographically significant coronary artery narrowing (greater than 50%) showed a much lower increase in myocardial blood flow distal to the stenosis than did those without disease or with insignificant lesions. As with radiolabeled particle studies, the presence of reduced regional myocardial blood flow (as measured by ^{133}Xe washout) in areas of abnormal wall motion suggests scarred and nonviable myocardium (See, Holman, et al., 1979). Abnormal wall motion without reduced regional myocardial blood flow suggests that the region is composed mainly of ischemic muscle rather than scar.

The ^{133}Xe technique has also been used to evaluate the success of aortocoronary bypass surgery (Goldberg, Crawley, et al., 1975; Korbuly, Formanek, et al., 1975). Both the area of myocardium that is perfused by a venous graft and the regional myocardial perfusion rates can be derived after ^{133}Xe injection into the graft.

Limitations

Like the radiolabeled particle technique, ^{133}Xe is absolutely dependent upon coronary catheterization; it has the additional disadvantages of requiring longer catheterization, greater data processing time, and a gamma camera in the catheterization laboratory. The computer analysis of the multiple ^{133}Xe washout curves, however, provides more quantitative information concerning the myocardial circulation than do the static, qualitative images obtained after injection of radiolabeled albumin particles. In addition, the ability to estimate regional myocardial blood flow both at rest and during such interventions as atrial pacing can permit an accurate assessment of the significance of a coronary artery lesion. Limitations of the ^{133}Xe techniques are related to methodological problems with the tracer (including short shelf life), the scintillation camera system, and anatomic and physiologic considerations (namely, the nonuniformity of blood flow that characterizes coronary artery disease); these limitations have been discussed in detail in excellent reviews by Cannon, Weiss, et al. (1977) and by Klocke (1976, 1983).

References

Ashburn, W. L.; Braunwald, E.; Simon, A. L., et al. 1971. Myocardial perfusion imaging with radioactive labeled particles injected directly into the coronary circulation of patients with coronary artery disease. *Circulation* 44:851–65.

Bulkley, B. H.; Rouleau, J. R.; Whitaker, J. Q., et al. 1977. The use of [201]thallium for myocardial perfusion imaging into sarcoid heart disease. *Chest* 72:27–32.

Cannon, P. J.; Dell, R. B.; and Dwyer, E. M., Jr. 1972a. Measurement of regional myocardial perfusion in man with 133 xenon and a scintillation camera. *J. Clin. Invest.* 51:964–77.

———. 1972b. Regional myocardial perfusion rates in patients with coronary artery disease. *J. Clin. Invest.* 51:978–94.

Cannon, P. J.; Haft, H. I.; and Johnson, B. M. 1969. Visual assessment of regional myocardial perfusion using radioactive xenon and scintillation photography. *Circulation* 40:277–88.

Cannon, P. J.; Schmidt, D. H.; Weiss, M. B., et al. 1975. The relationship between regional myocardial perfusion at rest and arteriographic lesions in patients with coronary atherosclerosis. *J. Clin. Invest.* 56:1442–54.

Cannon, P. J.; Weiss, M. B.; and Casarella, W. J. 1976. Studies of regional myocardial blood flow: Results in patients with left anterior descending coronary artery disease. *Semin. Nucl. Med.* 6:279–303.

Cannon, P. J.; Weiss, M. B.; and Sciacca, R. R. 1977. Myocardial blood flow in coronary artery disease: Studies at rest and during stress with inert gas washout techniques. *Prog. Cardiovasc. Dis.* 20:95-120.

Dwyer, E. M., Jr.; Dell, R. B.; and Cannon, P. J. 1973. Regional myocardial blood flow in patients with residual anterior and inferior transmural infarction. *Circulation* 48:924-35.

Endo, M.; Yamazaki, T.; Konno, S., et al. 1970. Direct diagnosis of human myocardial ischemia using ^{131}I-MAA via the selective coronary catheter. *Am. Heart J.* 80:498-506.

Goldberg, A. D.; Crawley, J. C. W.; Raftery, E. B., et al. 1975. Myocardial blood flowing saphenous vein bypass surgery. *Circulation* 51:215-19.

Gould, K. L.; Hamilton, G. W.; Lipscomb, K., et al. 1974. Method for assessing stress induced regional malperfusion during coronary arteriography: Experimental validation and clinical application. *Am. J. Cardiol.* 34:557-64.

Gould, K. L.; Lipscomb, K.; and Hamilton, G. W. 1974. A physiologic basis for assessing critical coronary stenosis: Instantaneous response and regional distribution during coronary hyperemia as measures of coronary flow reserve. *Am. J. Cardiol.* 33:87-94.

Grames, G. M.; Jansen, C.; Gander, M. P., et al. 1974. Safety of the direct coronary injection of radiolabelled particles. *J. Nucl. Med.* 15:2-6.

Hamilton, G. W.; Murray, J. A.; Lapin, E., et al. 1975. Evaluation of myocardial perfusion by direct injection of radioactive particles following coronary surgery. In *Coronary artery medicine and surgery: Concepts and controversies*, edited by J. C. Norman, 860-67. New York: Appleton-Century-Crofts.

Hamilton, G. W.; Ritchie, J. L.; Allen, D., et al. 1975. Myocardial perfusion imaging with ^{99m}Tc or [113m]In macroaggregated albumin: Correlation of the perfusion image with clinical, angiographic, surgical and histological findings. *Am. Heart J.* 89:708-15.

Holman, B. L.; Adams, D. F.; Jewitt, D., et al. 1974. Measuring regional myocardial blood flow with ^{133}Xe and the Anger camera. *Radiology* 112:99-107.

Horwitz, L. D.; Curry, G. C.; Parkey, R. W., et al. 1974. Differentiation of physiologically significant coronary artery lesions by coronary blood flow measurements during isoproterenol infusion. *Circulation* 49:55-62.

Hutchins, G. W.; Bulkley, B. H.; Ridolfi, R. L., et al. 1977. Correlation of coronary arteriograms and left ventriculograms with postmortem studies. *Circulation* 56:32-37.

Jansen, C.; Judkins, M. P.; Grames, G. M., et al. 1973. Myocardial perfusion color scintigraphy with MAA. *Radiology* 109:369-80.

Kirk, G. A.; Jansen, C.; and Judkins, M. P. 1977. Particulate myocardial perfusion scintigraphy: Its clinical usefulness in evaluation of coronary artery disease. *Semin. Nucl. Med.* 7:67–84.

Klocke, F. J. 1976. Coronary blood flow in man. *Prog. Cardiovasc. Dis.* 19:117–66.

———. 1983. Measurements of coronary blood flow and degree of stenosis: Current clinical implications and continuing uncertainties. *J. Am. Coll. Cardiol.* 1:31–41.

Korbuly, D. E.; Formanek, A.; Gypser, G., et al. 1975. Regional myocardial blood flow measurements before and after coronary bypass surgery. *Circulation* 52:38–45.

Kostuk, W. J. 1977. Myocardial perfusion assessed by direct coronary arterial injection of radiolabelled particles. In *Atherosclerosis: Metabolic, morphologic and clinical aspects.* Vol. 82, *Advances in experimental medicine and biology*, edited by G. W. Manning, 130–33. New York: Plenum Press.

Kostuk, W. J.; and Chamberlain, M. J. 1976a. Myocardial perfusion abnormalities in patients with cardiomyopathy. In *Microcirculation*, vol. 1, edited by J. Grayson and W. Zingg, 303–5. New York: Plenum Press.

———. 1976b. Myocardial perfusion defects in patients with valvular heart disease. In *Microcirculation*, vol. 1, edited by J. Grayson and W. Zingg, 301–2. New York: Plenum Press.

———. 1977. Predictive value of myocardial perfusion imaging for aorto-coronary bypass surgery. *Can. J. Surg.* 20:112–17.

Maseri, A.; and Mancini, P. 1972. The evaluation of regional myocardial perfusion in man by scintillation camera computer system. In *Myocardial blood flow in man*, edited by A. Maseri, 219–30. Torino: Minerva Medica.

Maseri, A.; L'Abbate, A.; Pesola, A., et al. 1977. Regional myocardial perfusion in patients with atherosclerotic coronary artery disease, at rest and during angina pectoris induced by tachycardia. *Circulation* 55:423–33.

Mundth, E. D.; and Austen, W. G. 1975. Surgical measures for coronary artery disease. *N. Engl. J. Med.* 293:13–19.

Poe, N. D.; Eber, L. M.; Norman, A. S., et al. 1977. Myocardial images in non-acute coronary and non-coronary heart disease. *J. Nucl. Med.* 18:18–23.

Ritchie, J. L.; Hamilton, G. W.; Gould, K. L., et al. 1975. Myocardial imaging with indium-113m and technetium-99m-macroaggregated albumin: New procedure for identification of stress-induced regional ischemia. *Am. J. Cardiol.* 35:380–89.

Roberts, W. C.; and Ferrans, V. J. 1974. Pathological aspects of certain cardiomyopathies. *Circ. Res.* 35:128–44.

Schmidt, D. H.; Weiss, M. B.; Casarella, W. J., et al. 1976. Regional myocardial perfusion during atrial pacing in patients with coronary artery disease. *Circulation* 53:807–19.

See, J. R.; Holman, B. L.; Adams, D. F., et al. 1979. Significance of reduced regional myocardial blood flow in asynergic areas evaluated with intervention ventriculography: Results of studies combining washout of xenon-133 and post extrasystolic potentiation. *Am. J. Cardiol.* 43:179–85.

Weller, D. A.; Adolph, R. J.; Wellman, H. N., et al. 1972. Myocardial perfusion scintigraphy after intracoronary injection of ^{99m}Tc-labeled human albumin microspheres: Toxicity and efficacy for detecting myocardial infarction in dogs; preliminary results in man. *Circulation* 46:963–75.

7 Radionuclide Angiography in Coronary Artery Disease

Peter R. McLaughlin, M.D.

Associate Director, Cardiovascular Unit, and
   Co-Director, Nuclear Cardiology Laboratory
Toronto General Hospital

Associate Professor
University of Toronto
Toronto, Ontario, Canada

Since Zaret and coworkers first described gated radionuclide angiography (Zaret, Strauss, et al., 1971), radioisotopes have become increasingly important in the noninvasive assessment of right and left ventricular function in patients with coronary disease. Ashburn and Schelbert subsequently showed that the single pass technique gave an accurate measure of the left ventricular ejection fraction (Schelbert, Verba, et al., 1975). In 1977, Burow and coworkers described the application of multiple gating to equilibrium radionuclide angiography in patients with suspected coronary artery disease. This important advance in computer software allows the physician to measure the ventricular ejection fraction and to visualize wall motion in more than one view, and serially if desired. Because this method is compatible with standard gamma cameras and with the automated software packages in relatively small computers, it is now widely used around the world.

In 1977, Borer and colleagues first illustrated the importance of assessing left ventricular function during exercise with radionuclide angiography. The response of the left ventricle to exercise has important diagnostic and therapeutic implications in assessing the efficacy of drug and surgical treatment. Finally, radionuclide angiography has given us a glimpse of the right ventricle and is allowing us to assess the effect of exercise and drugs on its function. This chapter will discuss the applications and limitations of radionuclide angiography, particularly in patients with coronary disease.

METHODS

The important parameters of ventricular function that can be assessed by radionuclide angiography include ejection fraction, wall motion, volume, and filling and emptying indices. These parameters can be determined both by first pass and gated equilibrium techniques, which are based on different principles. In the first pass technique, 10 to 20 mCi of radioactive technetium (^{99m}Tc) are injected as a bolus into a peripheral vein, with the patient positioned under the scintillation camera in the anterior view. Over the next 30 seconds, counts are continuously recorded and displayed as a function of time (time-activity curve) as the bolus passes through the right ventricle, lung fields, left ventricle, and into the aorta. Each systole and diastole is accompanied by a change in the ventricular count activity, which is proportional to changes in blood volume in the cavity. The time-activity curve for the ventricles appears as a series of peaks and troughs, each representing one ventricular contraction and relaxation. Since there is a lapse of several seconds while the ^{99m}Tc passes through the lung fields, the right and left ventricular time-activity curves can be temporally separated on subsequent computer analysis. Ejection fraction can be calculated accurately using the average ventricular "peak" count as end-diastole and "trough" counts as end-systoles, after correcting for residual background activity in the lung fields. The ejection fraction is calculated from the formula (counts are background corrected):

$$\text{Ejection fraction} = \frac{\text{End-diastolic counts} - \text{End-systolic counts}}{\text{End-diastolic counts}}$$

The summed time-activity curve for each ventricle can be displayed as a scintigraphic movie to delineate regional wall motion. Volumes have been calculated by tracing end-diastolic and end-systolic silhouettes and applying the geometric formula of Sandler and Dodge.

With the gated equilibrium study, ^{99m}Tc is labeled to red blood cells by an in-vivo labeling method, and for several hours it becomes an intravascular tracer. After equilibrium is reached in the blood pool (within a few minutes of injection of the ^{99m}Tc), the scintillation camera is positioned over the precordium in multiple views. Counts are recorded from the cardiac blood pool and fed into a computer with a simultaneous ECG signal. Using the R-wave as a trigger, the computer divides the cardiac cycle into a number of "frames," from 15 to 60 per cycle (Figure 7-1). The computer stores blood pool counts corresponding to each time frame in a different memory area. Over approximately 300 cycles, an image of the ventricular blood pools is accumulated for each time frame, proceeding from end-diastole through systole and back to end-diastole. Replaying these frame images in an endless loop movie format yields a simultaneous right and left ventricular angiogram and allows one to analyze regional wall motion in the different views recorded. Ejection fraction can be calculated accurately by selecting the end-diastolic and end-systolic frames and quantitating the counts within the ventricular silhouette. After determining the background contribution to the ventricular counts, ejection

ECG Gated Angiography

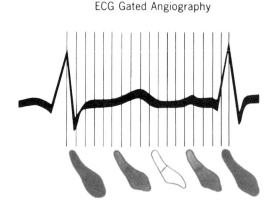

Figure 7-1 The principle of ECG gating for equilibrium blood pool angiograms.

fraction is determined by the formula used for the first pass technique. The left anterior oblique view (Figure 7-2) is used for ejection fraction determinations because this view provides the best spatial separation of the ventricles. Several commercial computer systems provide semiautomated programs for ejection fraction analysis. In addition to ejection fraction and regional wall motion, several investigators have attempted to quantitate absolute ventricular volumes from the gated equilibrium study.

VIEWS AND INTERPRETATION

The standard views obtained with the gated equilibrium study are the 45° (with slight caudal angulation) and 70° left anterior oblique and anterior or right anterior oblique (Figure 7-3). Figure 7-4 illustrates the left and right ventricular segments visualized in the two 45° oblique views. Systolic wall motion of each segment may be graded subjectively as "normal," "hypokinetic" (reduced motion), "akinetic" (absent motion), or "dyskinetic" (paradoxical outward systolic motion). In systems where both black-and-white and color displays are interchangeable, it is useful to display the ventricles in both formats. The monochromatic display is more useful in assessing wall motion, while the color display, by drawing the viewer's eye to the motion of the blood volume, provides a visual display

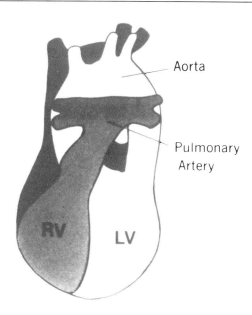

Figure 7-2 The left anterior oblique view of a gated radionuclide angiogram.

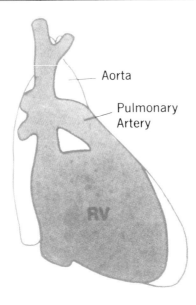

Figure 7-3 The right anterior oblique view of a gated radionuclide angiogram.

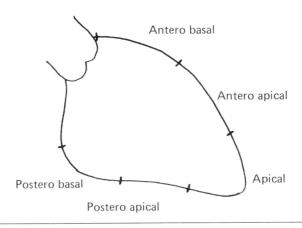

Figure 7-4 Schematic illustration of the segments in the right and left anterior oblique views.

of volume change (ejection fraction). In our laboratory we prefer the black-and-white display for all routine studies. Figure 7-5 illustrates an end-diastolic and end-systolic frame from such a patient with normal left and right ventricular function. All segments demonstrated normal homogeneous inward motion in a synchronous manner.

As the interpreter assesses regional wall motion in the gated equilibrium study, he or she must be wary of the segments affected by superimposition. In the anterior or right anterior oblique view, the basal segments of the left ventricle may be obscured by the body and outflow tract of the right ventricle, especially in subjects with right ventricular enlargement. In the left anterior oblique view, in studies recorded with a standard parallel-hole collimator, the upper margins of the left ventricle may be partially obscured by the left atrium. However, most of the ventricle can be easily appreciated, and use of the slant-hole collimator with a 15°–30° caudal tilt provides even better separation of the left atrium and ventricle.

The right ventricle may be visualized by itself only in the left anterior oblique view, which provides an "end-on" view of both ventricles. Normal anterior and inferior walls show uniform systolic inward motion, although appreciably less than the left ventricular segments. The upper margin of the free wall of the anterior right ventricle may be partially obscured by the right atrium at end-systole when the atrium is maximally filled. Viewing the real-time ciné replay usually allows one to visualize the atrioventricular groove separation, and, again, a caudal tilt of the camera or collimator may help.

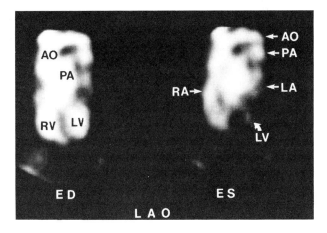

Figure 7-5 An end-diastolic and end-systolic frame from a normal gated radionuclide angiogram in the left anterior oblique view.

VALIDATION AND LIMITATIONS

Because contrast angiography at cardiac catheterization remains the standard for left ventricular volumes and ejection fraction, radionuclide angiography has been validated by correlation with contrast studies. For both the gated and first pass methods, a number of investigators (Van Dyke, Anger, et al., 1972; Berman, Salel, et al., 1975; Schelbert, Verba, et al., 1975; Burow, Strauss, et al., 1977; Marshall, Berger, et al., 1977; Slutsky, Curtis, et al., 1979) have demonstrated excellent correlations for ejection fraction with correlation coefficients ranging from 0.80 to 0.95. Early attempts to determine left ventricular volumes by radionuclide angiography used area-length formulas applied to tracings of end-systolic and end-diastolic frames. Although this method gave satisfactory correlations with volumes calculated from contrast angiograms, it has significant disadvantages. In ventricles with nonellipsoid shapes the area-length formula has intrinsic errors, and accurate border recognition is difficult in the radionuclide angiogram. More recently, Slutsky and coworkers described a new method in which volumes are determined from background-corrected left ventricular counts calibrated with counts in a sample of the patient's blood (Slutsky, Gordon, et al., 1979). Refinements and modifications in this technique (Links, Becker, et al., 1983) constitute a genuine improvement because they eliminate the errors introduced by geometric formulas. Because the counts at the periphery of the ventricle are small in relation to the central volume, the precision of border recognition is not as critical as with the area-length method, and hence the error is again reduced.

Regional wall motion can be assessed qualitatively with a reasonable degree of accuracy by radionuclide angiography. Quantification of regional wall motion abnormalities has been attempted with both chord shortening analysis (Bodenheimer, Banka, et al., 1978b) and regional ejection fraction analysis. Chord shortening techniques depend upon accurate border recognition, which again introduces the possibility of significant error. Regional ejection fraction analysis, which is based on changes in regional count, is sounder. In this method a centroid (mathematical center of the count volume) is chosen and radii or chords are extended to the silhouette, dividing the ventricle into a number of regions. Counts in each region are compared in the end-diastolic and end-systolic frames to calculate regional ejection fraction. The alternative method for regional ejection fraction divides the ventricle into a number of rectangles to which similar count analysis is applied (Maddox, Wynne, et al., 1979). However, both methods have limitations.

In studies recorded with standard collimators, the essential difficulty is the accurate identification of the true end-systolic centroid from which to draw the radii or chords. For example, an aneurysmal region that paradoxically expands during systole would artefactually draw the count "centroid" to the dyskinetic segment, reducing the regional ejection fraction of opposing normal segments and increasing that of the abnormal segment. (Choosing to use the centroid or rectangle for the end-systolic frame in the same location as for the end-diastolic frame would not account for shifts in the position of the ventricle as it contracts.) Hence, errors are present in either method.

The introduction of tomographic angiography using a rotating camera overcomes many of these objections because an ejection fraction can be determined for each "slice" from base to apex. This technique will be covered in more detail later. It should be noted that regional wall-motion analysis in the contrast angiogram is also hampered by many limitations and errors, but these do not necessarily invalidate its clinical usefulness.

In addition to the problems of regional wall-motion analysis, both the first pass and gated equilibrium studies have certain basic limitations. Table 7-1 compares the relative advantages and disadvantages of these two methods. The advantages of the gated equilibrium method include its ability to record different views and several studies before and after an intervention with a single dose of ^{99m}Tc, to allow longer counting times and hence better resolution for wall-motion analysis, and its compatibility with the standard single crystal camera. Its disadvantages are the length of time required to record a study (five to 15 minutes), the difficulty in analysis of wall motion in the right anterior oblique or anterior view as a result of superimposition, and the necessity of a stable rhythm to provide an accurate ECG trigger.

Table 7-2 compares the limitations of contrast and radionuclide angiography. The major advantage of the radionuclide technique is that it provides a safe, accurate, noninvasive method for assessment of ventricular function that is associated with low patient radiation. The radionuclide technique overcomes the error in the geometric formula for volume deter-

Table 7-1 Comparison of single pass and gated blood pool radionuclide angiography

Single pass	*Gated blood pool*
30 seconds to record	2–5 minutes to record
Independent of rhythm	Stable rhythm required
Good separation of RV and LV in either RAO or LAO	Good separation of RV and LV in LAO view only
Only one view per injection; only one study per injection	Biplane and multiple studies with one injection
Limited counting times for resolution of wall motion	Longer counting time may improve resolution of wall motion
Multicrystal camera optimal	Standard single crystal camera used

Notes: RV = right ventricle; LV = left ventricle; LAO = left anterior oblique; RAO = right anterior oblique.

Table 7-2 Comparison of radionuclide and contrast angiography

Radionuclide	Contrast
Noninvasive: vein injection only	Invasive: requires catheterization
Can be done at bedside with mobile camera	Patient must be moved
No morbidity	Morbidity of catheterization
Lower radiation: 150–400 m rads whole body	Higher radiation: approximately 500–1000 m rads for catheterization and angiography (mean body dose)
Accurate ejection fraction	Accurate ejection fraction in normal ventricle; possible error with large or segmentally diseased ventricle
Exercise angiograms readily done	Exercise angiograms difficult
Background count correction may result in error	No background error
Superimposition of RV and LV in RAO gated study, superimposition of atria on ventricular silhouettes	No superimposition with selective ventricular opacification
Absolute volume developmental	Absolute volume can be calculated
Valvular insufficiency developmental	Valvular insufficiency can be assessed
Equipment costly	Equipment costly

mination that is applied to the contrast angiogram to derive volumes and ejection fraction. This formula assumes an ellipsoid ventricular shape, an assumption that is false in the large or segmentally diseased ventricle. An important advantage of the radionuclide angiogram is its portability. The mobile scintillation camera can be taken directly to the acutely ill patient for serial bedside studies. Finally, the radionuclide angiogram permits one to study serially the effects of exercise on ventricular function—a much more difficult task with the repeat contrast angiograms during exercise in the catheterization laboratory.

The radionuclide angiogram has a number of limitations when compared to contrast angiography. Its accuracy depends in part upon the ability to determine consistently the contribution of the pulmonary and mediastinal background to the ventricular counts. Any difference in pulmonary flow between the assumed background area and the true background regions in front and behind the ventricle will introduce an error. Similarly, small changes in the choice of the background region, particularly in its proximity to the ventricular silhouette, can result in significant differences in background counts and hence in the calculation of ejection fractions. (Although the semiautomated methods for choosing background areas may make the error more consistent, some variability is inevitable.) As mentioned, superimposition of the atria and ventricles in the right anterior oblique and anterior views in the gated study interferes with wall-motion analysis of the individual ventricles. Since the left or right ventricle is selectively injected with contrast medium during catheterization, no such superimposition impedes analysis of the contrast angiogram. Volumes can be calculated from contrast angiograms, with the limitations noted above, while the radionuclide angiography volume determination is still undergoing development and refinement. In addition, the contrast angiogram allows assessment of valvular insufficiency. Since all the atria, ventricles, and aorta are in equilibrium during the gated radionuclide study, it is difficult to visualize retrograde flow. Although some preliminary work has been done to quantitate aortic and atrial regurgitation with radionuclide angiography (Rigo, Alderson, et al., 1979), further studies are required. Finally, it should be noted that the scintillation camera and computer system together cost from $130,000 to over $200,000, depending upon the sophistication of the equipment. Angiographic equipment, of course, costs even more; hence, cost becomes a limitation for both systems.

NORMAL STUDY AND INTERVENTIONS

Rest

As mentioned earlier, the important parameters of ventricular function assessed by radionuclide angiography are ejection fraction, regional wall motion, volume, and filling and emptying indices. The normal left ventricular ejection fraction at rest is greater than 0.50 in most laboratories and may range up to 0.75. Normal variability, technique, and the system used explain this broad range. Left ventricular ejection fractions less than 0.50 are considered abnormal.

The normal right ventricular ejection fraction at rest is lower than the left and ranges from 0.35 to 0.65. The right ventricle matches the left ventricular stroke volume by functioning at a higher end-diastolic volume. Until quantitative regional wall-motion analysis becomes more widely accepted, the clinician will continue to use qualitative analysis in daily practice. Normal wall motion, whether at rest or after an intervention, is a homogeneous inward systolic movement, as opposed to hypokinesis, akinesis, or dyskinesis. Changes in ventricular volume from rest to exercise will be discussed.

Exercise

Patients with coronary disease without previous infarction often have normal ventricular function at rest. Just as they are free of symptoms at rest and experience angina or dyspnea with exertion, exercise may provoke profound changes in left ventricular function as a consequence of transient myocardial ischemia. Thus the assessment of the left and right ventricles at rest and during exercise has become useful in assessing patients with suspected coronary disease (Rerych, Scholz, et al., 1978; Berger, Johnstone, et al., 1979; Berger, Reduto, et al., 1979; Borer, Kent, et al., 1979; Frischknecht, Steele, et al., 1979; Jengo, Oren, et al., 1979; Johnson, McCarthy, et al., 1979).

Figure 7-6 illustrates the normal increase of the left and right ventricular ejection fraction during exercise in a 24-year-old man with no evidence of heart disease. The usual normal response to exercise is an increase in ejection from zero to 20%. In our laboratory, we have opted to maintain a higher specificity at the expense of a reduced sensitivity. We accept a decrease in exercise ejection fraction of 5% or greater as an indication of definitely abnormal left ventricular reserve; a decrease of zero to 5% as borderline but not abnormal; and an increase as within normal limits. However, many laboratories would judge any decrease as abnormal, and others, any increase less than 5% as abnormal. As seen in Figure 7-6, the right and left ventricular responses parallel each other as exercise progresses. In our own early experience of 17 control patients with no clinical evidence of coronary disease, two had either a flat or a slightly decreasing left ventricular ejection fraction response during exercise. Abnormal stress global and regional ejection fractions have been noted by other investigators in a small percentage of "normal" patients with normal coronary arteriograms (Bodenheimer, Banka, et al., 1979; Gibbons, Lee, et al., 1981), and Jones and coworkers have shown that with age the left ven-

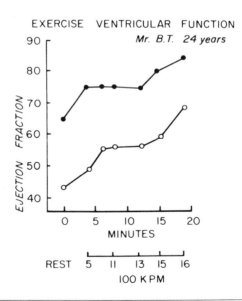

Figure 7-6   The normal right and left ventricular ejection fraction response to exercise.

tricular ejection fraction response to exercise decreases (Port, Cobb, et al., 1980). Whether this represents normal variation or preclinical heart disease remains to be determined. Of interest, Berger demonstrated abnormal left ventricular reserve (less than a 5% increase with exercise) in 12 of 31 patients with normal coronary arteries but ischemic exercise ECGs and chest pain (Berger, Sands, et al., 1981).

The practical importance of these studies for the clinician is that a fall in left ventricular ejection fraction with exercise is not specific for coronary artery disease. A decrease greater than 5% means that left ventricular reserve is abnormally impaired, whether it be from coronary artery or other disease such as cardiomyopathy. A decrease of zero to 5% may mean mild impairment of reserve, but may also be a variant of normal in a few subjects.

The changes in left ventricular volume during exercise are also of considerable interest. Using the technique for determining absolute volumes described earlier, Slutsky and coworkers studied volume changes during exercise (Slutsky, Karliner, et al., 1979a, b). In their group of 10 normal men, no significant change in end-diastolic volume from rest to peak supine exercise was observed. These results can be contrasted with our own experience with 19 normal controls in whom there was a 9% increase (P<0.05) in left ventricular end-diastolic relative volume at peak supine exercise (Bar-Shlomo, Druck, et al., 1982). In this study we made no attempt to quantitate absolute volumes in milliliters, but rather assessed "relative" volume changes by comparing end-diastolic and end-systolic counts at peak exercise to rest. Willerson and coworkers reported similar results (Poliner, Dehmer, et al., 1979).

The effect of posture on ejection fraction and ventricular volume is important, both at rest and during exercise. Most investigators have used supine bicycle exercise because of its ease of application, but some have studied volume changes in the upright position. Jones and coworkers showed a slight increase in end-diastolic volume at peak upright exercise in normal controls, although volumes were measured by applying area-length formulas to the traced silhouettes. Willerson and coworkers compared upright and supine exercise in normal subjects (Poliner, Dehmer, et al., 1979). They also found an increase in end-diastolic volume at peak exercise in both the supine and upright positions. However, the end-diastolic volume was significantly greater in the supine position, reflecting greater venous return. The resting ejection fraction was greater in the upright position and showed a larger increase in percentage with exercise than the corresponding supine values. For these reasons, the patient's position must be kept in mind in the interpretation of one's own data and those of others.

Finally, the type of exercise deserves comment. Dynamic work, such as bicycling, is the most common type of stress applied for radionuclide angiography. Most patients experience symptoms during dynamic exercise and the physiologic changes in heart rate, blood pressure, and venous return are greater with this type of exercise. However, Helfant and co-workers have also used isometric hand-grip exercise as a stress with radionuclide angiography (Bodenheimer, Banka, et al., 1978a). They showed that abnormal left ventricular function can be provoked by hand grip. Its advantages are its simplicity and absence of motion artefact, but the associated physiologic changes tend to be less than with dynamic leg exercise, and hence it may be less potent in provoking ischemia. Several investigators have also used the cold pressor test, although it appears to be of limited usefulness.

Recently, increasing attention has turned to the assessment of diastolic function of the left ventricle from the rates of filling of the ventricle. These data can be obtained from the slope of the diastolic portion of the time-activity curve, i.e., from the bottom of the trough at end-systole back up the curve to end-diastole. These filling indices relate in part to diastolic compliance, which is altered in many disease states, such as in hypertension with left ventricular hypertrophy and in ischemia of the ventricle. Radionuclide angiography provides a means of assessing the effect of drug therapy on diastolic function, but the practical relevance of this to the clinician remains to be seen.

MYOCARDIAL ISCHEMIA

As is well known, exercise may induce myocardial ischemia in patients with coronary disease. Radionuclide angiography provides a method of looking at another manifestation of myocardial ischemia—ventricular dysfunction. Figure 7-7 shows the left ventricular response to exercise in a 64-year-old man with a 90% narrowing of the left anterior descending artery and 100% occlusion of the right coronary artery. The ejection fraction was normal at rest (0.65) but declined markedly to 0.38 as the patient achieved only a mild load (300 kpm) before experiencing angina. During recovery the angina subsided and the ejection fraction returned to normal. When the real-time replay of the angiogram was viewed, wall motion was normal at rest. At peak exercise the septal and inferior segments of the left ventricle became severely hypokinetic as a result of exercise-induced ischemia, and returned to normal during recovery. Hence the ejection fraction response and appearance of new regional wall motion abnormalities can represent a noninvasive method for detecting or assessing the significance of coronary artery lesions. If exercise radionuclide angiography is to be useful in detecting suspected coronary disease, it must satisfy two criteria: first, it must have a satisfactory sensitivity, specificity, and predictive accuracy; second, it must provide useful diagnostic information that cannot be obtained by other, simpler noninvasive tests such as the exercise electrocardiogram.

A number of investigators have reported results of exercise radionuclide angiography in the detection of coronary artery disease (Rerych, Scholz, et al., 1978; Berger, Reduto, et al., 1979; Borer, Kent, et al.,

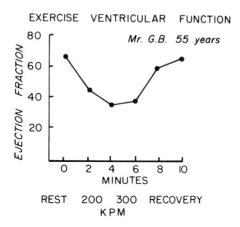

Figure 7-7 An abnormal exercise left ventricular ejection fraction response secondary to exercise-induced ischemia in a patient with two-vessel coronary disease.

1979; Caldwell, Sorensen, et al., 1979; Jengo, Oren, et al., 1979; Kirshenbaum, Okada, et al., 1979; Verani, Del Ventura, et al., 1979). These results in 427 patients have been summarized by Okada, Boucher, et al. (1980) and are compared to exercise ECG results in Table 7-3.

A new regional wall motion abnormality on exercise is the most specific indicator of coronary disease (100%), but has a sensitivity of only approximately 75%. An increase in the exercise ejection fraction of at least 5% is more sensitive (87%) but less specific (93%). Clinically, when one uses both of these indicators together, the sensitivity approximates 87% with a specificity of 92%. These limits are quite acceptable for clinical practice if the test is applied wisely.

For example, if the test is applied to a population with a disease prevalence of 50%—that is, patients considered to be "suspicious" for coronary disease by the examining physician—the resulting positive predictive accuracy would be 92% and the negative predictive accuracy 88% (Table 7-4). In this case, a positive or abnormal result means a 92% likelihood of disease, while a negative result means an 88% likelihood of being normal. On the other hand, if the same test is applied to an asymptomatic general population of late-middle-aged males, with a disease prevalence of 10%, the positive predictive accuracy would be 57% and the negative predictive accuracy, 1%. In this case, a negative test would be very useful in ruling out the likelihood of disease, while a positive test would mean only a moderate probability of disease.

In considering the results of these studies, a number of points should be kept in mind. The studies excluded patients with heart disease other

Table 7-3 Reported results of blood pool angiographic exercise test

Year	Principal investigator (location)	Method	Patients (n)	RWM		EF		RWM + EF		Ex ECG	
				Sens	Spec	Sens	Spec	Sens	Spec	Sens	Spec
1978	Rerych (Durham)	Erect first pass	60	24/30	—	29/30	27/30	29/30	27/30	23/30	—
1979	Borer (Bethesda)	Supine gated	84	59/63	21/21	56/63	21/21	60/63	21/21	43/63	20/21
1979	Berger (New Haven)	Supine or erect first pass	73	28/60	13/13	44/60	13/13	52*/60	13/13	33/60	13/13
1979	Jengo (Torrance)	Erect first pass	19	11/11	8/8	11/11	8/8	11/11	8/8	7/11	—
1979	Caldwell (Seattle)	Supine + erect	39	—	—	31/33	4/6	—	—	—	—
1979	Borer (Bethesda)	Supine gated	53	—	—	—	—	40/43	10/10	—	—
1979	Verani (Houston)	Supine gated	38	—	—	—	—	11/21	16/17	—	—
1980	Kirshenbaum (Boston)	Supine gated	61	—	—	—	—	38/50	6/11	32/50	11/11
Total			427	122/164 0.73	42/42 1.00	171/197 0.87	73/78 0.93	241/276 0.87	101/110 0.92	138/214 0.64	44/45 0.98

*Includes four patients with abnormalities at rest only.

Notes: EF = failure to increase ejection fraction by 5% with exercise; Ex ECG = abnormal exercise electrocardiogram; RWM = exercise-induced regional wall motion abnormality; Sens = sensitivity; Spec = specificity; — = data not reported.
Reproduced, with permission , from Okada, R. D.; Boucher, C. A.; Strauss, H. W., et al. 1980. *Am. J. Cardiol.* 46:1188-1204.

124

Table 7-4 Predictive accuracy of exercise radionuclide angiography*

A. *Disease prevalence = 50%*

Exercise radionuclide angiographic results	True coronary disease	No coronary disease	Total
+	44	4	48
-	6	46	52
Total	50	50	100

Positive predictive accuracy = 44/48 = 92%
Negative predictive accuracy = 46/52 = 88%

B. *Disease prevalence = 10%*

Exercise radionuclide angiographic results	True coronary disease	No coronary disease	Total
+	9	7	16
-	1	83	84
Total	10	90	100

Positive predictive accuracy = 9/16 = 57%
Negative predictive accuracy = 83/84 = 99%

*Using a sensitivity of 87% and specificity of 92%.

than coronary atherosclerosis. If those with valvular disease or cardio-myopathies were included in the normal coronary artery group, we would see many more abnormal global ejection fraction responses to exercise, although only infrequent abnormal regional ejection fraction responses. Also, the clinician should remember that the end-point of these noninvasive tests is a physiologic abnormality, myocardial ischemia, for which there is no true standard. Instead, results are compared to an anatomic abnormality, a narrowing in a coronary arteriogram that gives no information about coronary flow. Thus, some "false negative" noninvasive tests may be attributable not to the failure of the test to detect existing ischemia, but rather to the fact that a particular stress applied to a particular lesion did not produce ischemia. The other difficulty is that although coronary arteriography is the most reliable standard available it is also an imperfect test that gives rise to some false negatives in patients with coronary disease and coronary spasm.

In addition to detection of coronary disease, exercise radionuclide angiography can be used to assess the functional significance of coronary artery lesions, much as thallium-201 and exercise electrocardiography have proved useful. For example, it is not uncommon to find on coronary arteriography a "50% lesion," the significance of which is not clear. The demonstration of exercise-induced ischemia distal to such a lesion can greatly assist in the management of the patient with slightly atypical pain or help to localize sites of ischemia before and after operation. The appearance of exercise-induced regional dysfunction would have the same significance as a new defect on an exercise thallium-201 study, indicating that a particular lesion is producing ischemia. Similarly, exercise radionuclide angiography may be useful in selected patients for assessing their response to antianginal therapy, an exercise rehabilitation program, coronary bypass surgery (Kent, Borer, et al., 1978), and other methods used in the treatment of coronary disease.

Although the data and concepts discussed so far have related to left ventricular function, radionuclide angiography also provides an excellent method of assessing right ventricular function. Until recently, the right ventricle received little attention in coronary artery disease, but the importance of right ventricular infarction has now been recognized and several investigators are studying the possibility of right ventricular ischemia during exercise.

Cannon and coworkers studied 37 patients at rest and during bicycle exercise, including 11 normal controls, 12 patients with significant proximal right coronary disease (involving the right ventricular blood supply), and 14 patients with distal right or other coronary vessel disease (Johnson, McCarthy, et al., 1979). These investigators found an abnormal, flat right ventricular ejection fraction response in patients with proximal right coronary disease, but a normal increase in patients with no involvement of the proximal right coronary artery. In contrast, in a group of 46 patients, Berger, Johnstone, et al. (1979) found that right ventricular performance was independent of proximal right coronary stenosis, but did relate to the left ventricular response. All patients with abnormal right ventricular reserve on exercise had abnormal left ventricular reserve, although some with normal right ventricular reserve did have an abnormal left ventricular response. They concluded that abnormal right ventricular reserve on exercise is common in patients with coronary disease, and the left ventricular response to exercise is the major determinant. Whether the mechanism is a direct ischemic effect because of involvement of its blood supply or a more indirect left ventricular effect, right ventricular function can deteriorate markedly during exercise in patients with coronary disease, which no doubt contributes to some of their symptoms. Maddahi, Wynne, et al. (1979) have further demonstrated that right ventricular ejection fraction can be equally well measured with gated equilibrium radionuclide angiography as with first pass studies, making right ventricular assessment more widely applicable.

In perspective, radionuclide angiography should not be viewed as the only or ideal noninvasive test for the investigation of a patient with known or suspected coronary artery disease. It is one of a number of sophisticated noninvasive tools available to the clinician. In most cases a careful history and physical examination, along with a resting ECG, will provide the information essential to the diagnosis. The exercise ECG is currently being used widely to assist in diagnosis and to assess functional capacity. The radionuclide angiogram adds a new dimension and gives a direct look at ventricular size and function. The angiogram is not necessary in all patients but is most useful when the clinician is aware of its proper use and limitations. The resting study may suffice in some patients, but for patients with symptoms it is highly desirable to visualize the ventricles during exericse.

ACUTE MYOCARDIAL INFARCTION

In recent years, considerable work has been done to characterize the clinical and hemodynamic variables of acute myocardial infarction. Until the advent of intracoronary streptokinase, only a few patients with acute infarction had cardiac catheterization and contrast left ventricular angiography. Thus, relatively little information about regional wall motion and ejection fractions has accompanied the clinical and hemodynamic data. The introduction of radionuclide angiography and the portable scintillation camera now allows the clinician to assess these patients with safety at their bedside. In addition to diagnostic and prognostic information, radionuclide angiography gives the physician a potentially important means of assessing the effects of drugs on ventricular function in acute infarction.

Schelbert, Henning, et al. (1976) first studied patients early and late (mean 20 months) after acute infarction, using single pass radionuclide angiography. These investigators showed that the ejection fraction often changes in the early postinfarct period and has prognostic importance for morbidity and mortality. Reduto, Berger, et al. (1978) similarly evaluated 31 patients with uncomplicated acute transmural myocardial infarction on four occasions during their hospitalization. They found that inferior infarction resulted in a reduction in right ventricular ejection fraction in one-half of the patients, while it was reduced in only one of 13 patients with anterior infarction. However, anterior infarction resulted in a more profound reduction in left ventricular function. In contrast to the early study of Schelbert, Henning, et al., they found no significant serial change in ejection fraction during the hospital course. However, there was close agreement with a later study by Schelbert and coworkers in which 37% of patients with inferior left ventricular infarction had right ventricular infarction with reduction of right ventricular ejection fraction (Tobinick, Schelbert, et al., 1978).

More recent studies by Morrison, Coromilas, et al. (1980) have suggested that radionuclide angiography may prove useful in the sizing of infarction. Battler, Slutsky, et al. (1980) and Wynne, Sayres, et al. (1980)

have also shown that radionuclide angiography, early after acute infarction, has important implications in determining late prognosis. In the study by Battler, Slutsky, et al. (1980), a global ejection fraction of <0.52 predicted a significant increase in combined mortality from congestive heart failure and mortality during the first year after infarction.

One of the important applications of radionuclide angiography following myocardial infarction is the detection of a left ventricular aneurysm. Several studies have now demonstrated the usefulness of this technique for the noninvasive visualization of both true and false aneurysms (Botvinick, Shames, et al., 1976; Friedman and Cantor, 1979; Froehlich, Falsetti, et al., 1980; Winzelberg, Miller, et al., 1980). Friedman recently demonstrated an overall accuracy rate of 96% for detection of aneurysm as compared to contrast angiography. The data available on detection of false aneurysms are based only on small patient numbers as yet; however, visualization of a large, usually posterior, paraventricular chamber with a narrow-necked connection to the ventricle is suggestive.

This clinically important application arises in the patient with known previous infarction who presents with congestive failure. Patients with a potentially resectable aneurysm can be selected for cardiac catheterization and possible surgery, while those with diffuse irreversible left ventricular dysfunction can be spared the invasive procedure.

In addition to these diagnostic studies, it is anticipated that considerable work will be done in the next few years to evaluate the effect of therapy on biventricular function in acute infarction. Data are needed on the effects of afterload and preload reducing agents, new inotropic drugs, coronary thrombolytic therapy, and mechanical assist devices to better evaluate their efficacy in acute infarction.

DRUGS AND CORONARY DISEASE

Although exercise is the most commonly used intervention under study, radionuclide angiography affords the opportunity to assess the effect of other interventions on left and right ventricular function. The capacity to study ventricular function serially has made the radionuclide angiogram an ideal method for assessing drug effects. It is not surprising that nitroglycerin and propranolol have received the most attention. Salel, Berman, et al. (1976) and Ritchie, Sorensen, et al. (1979) studied the effects of sublingual nitroglycerin on left ventricular dysfunction, and both groups of investigators demonstrated a reduction in end-diastolic volume and improvement in ejection fraction. The study conducted by Salel, Berman, et al. (1976) showed greater improvement in the group without ECG evidence of prior infarction.

Slutsky, Curtis, et al. (1979) compared the effect of nitroglycerin in patients at rest and during spontaneous angina. In patients free from pain, nitroglycerin produced an increase in ejection fraction six to eight minutes after ingestion, with an equal decrease in end-diastolic and end-systolic volume. These changes returned to baseline within one hour. During spontaneous angina, ejection fraction decreased, with a slight increase in end-diastolic volume and a marked increase in end-systolic volume. These changes were reversed after nitroglycerin administration and were associated with a drop in systolic pressure.

Ramanathan, Bodenheimer, et al. (1979) compared effects in patients with acute infarction and remote infarction. Regional contraction was improved by nitroglycerin in zones of acute infarction but not in zones of remote infarction. It was not clear whether the improved regional contraction was a result of improvement in contraction of viable muscle in the acutely infarcted zone, changes in infarct compliance, or an indirect result of improved contraction in noninfarcted areas.

Radionuclide angiography has been used to study the effects of propranolol. Zaret and coworkers studied 22 patients with stable coronary disease on chronic oral propranolol (Marshall, Berger, et al., 1978) and were unable to demonstrate any deleterious effects on resting left ventricular function. Borer, Bacharach, et al. (1978) showed a slight depression of resting ejection fraction by propranolol, but demonstrated that it protected against the exercise-induced deterioration of ejection fraction in patients with ischemic heart disease. This preservation of exercise ventricular function in coronary patients has been noted by other researchers (Battler, Ross, et al., 1979; Marshall, Wisenberg, et al., 1979), and probably reflects prevention of myocardial ischemia during exercise by propranolol.

These studies are only the first of many that will appear over the next two or three years providing new information on the effects of many commonly used cardiac drugs on left and right ventricular function.

TOMOGRAPHIC RADIONUCLIDE ANGIOGRAPHY

The principles of tomographic imaging and its application to thallium-201 imaging have been discussed in previous chapters. Vogel and coworkers (1979) described its application to radionuclide angiography using the seven-pinhole collimator. The technique of the gated equilibrium study was the same except that the seven-pinhole collimator was used in place of the standard parallel-hole collimator. After collection had been completed, the computer algorithm "reconstructed" the ventricle from apex to base in slices similar to the thallium-201 study. Gating provided an "angiogram" of each slice, and ejection fraction was calculated for each slice by the usual count analysis method. In this unique visualization of the left ventricle, all segments were seen without superimposition of other structures.

Similar methods could theoretically be used with the rotating gamma camera for single photon emission computed tomographic (SPECT) angiography. Since the algorithm could reconstruct the left ventricle in an isolated form, it appears possible that the ventricle could be displayed by itself in isolated global views rather than slices, eliminating the superimposition in the anterior and right anterior oblique views—a promising advance. As the software for gated radionuclide angiography using these cameras is developed, a more accurate reconstruction of both ventricles can be expected. At present there are practical limitations to SPECT angiography, and studies are needed to determine the limitations and clinical usefulness of the technique.

References

Bar-Shlomo, B. Z.; Druck, M. N.; Morch, J. E., et al. 1982. Left ventricular function in trained and untrained healthy subjects. *Circulation* 65:484–88.

Battler, A.; Ross, J.; Slutsky, R., et al. 1979. Improvement by oral propranolol of exercise-induced ischemic dysfunction in patients with coronary heart disease. Abstract, *Am. J. Cardiol.* 43:415.

Battler, A.; Slutsky, R.; Karliner, R., et al. 1980. Left ventricular ejection fraction and first third ejection fraction after acute myocardial infarction: Value for predicting mortality and morbidity. *Am. J. Cardiol.* 45:197–202.

Berger, H. J.; Johnstone, D. E.; Sands, J. M., et al. 1979. Response of right ventricular ejection fraction to upright bicycle exercise in coronary disease. *Circulation* 60:1292–1300.

Berger, H. J.; Reduto, L. A.; Johnstone, D. E., et al. 1979. Global and regional left ventricular response to bicycle exercise in coronary artery disease: Assessment by quantitative radionuclide angiography. *Am. J. Med.* 66:13–21.

Berger, H. J.; Sands, M. J.; Davies, R. A., et al. 1981. Exercise left ventricular performance in patients with chest pain, ischemic-appearing exercise electrocardiograms, and angiographically normal coronary arteries. *Ann. Intern. Med.* 94:186–91.

Berman, D. S.; Salel, A. F.; DeNardo, G. L., et al. 1975. Clinical assessment of left ventricular regional contraction patterns and ejection fraction by high-resolution gated scintigraphy. *J. Nucl. Med.* 16:865–74.

Bodenheimer, M. M.; Banka, V. S.; Fooshee, C. M., et al. 1978a. Detection of coronary heart disease using radionuclide determined regional ejection fraction at rest and during handgrip exercise: Correlation with coronary arteriography. *Circulation* 68:640–48.

———. 1978b. Quantitative radionuclide angiography in the right anterior oblique view: Comparison with contrast angiography. *Am. J. Cardiol.* 41:718–25.

———. 1979. Comparative sensitivity of the exercise electrocardiogram, thallium imaging and stress radionuclide angiography to detect the presence and severity of coronary heart disease. *Circulation* 60:1270–78.

Borer, J. S.; Bacharach, S. L.; Green, M. V., et al. 1977. Real-time radionuclide cineangiography in the noninvasive evaluation of global and regional left ventricular function at rest and during exercise in patients with coronary disease. *N. Engl. J. Med.* 296:839–44.

Borer, J. S.; Kent, K. M.; Bacharach, S. L., et al. 1979. Sensitivity, specificity and predictive accuracy of radionuclide cineangiography during exercise in patients with coronary artery disease: Comparison with exercise electrocardiography. *Circulation* 60:572–80.

Botvinick, E. H.; Shames, D.; Hutchinson, J. C., et al. 1976. Noninvasive diagnosis of a false left ventricular aneurysm with radioisotope gated cardiac blood pool imaging. *Am. J. Cardiol.* 37:1089–93.

Burow, R. D.; Strauss, H. W.; Singleton, R., et al. 1977. Analysis of left ventricular function from multiple gated acquisition cardiac blood pool imaging: Comparison to contrast angiography. *Circulation* 56:1024–28.

Caldwell, J.; Sorensen, S.; Ritchie, J., et al. 1979. Exercise radionuclide ventriculography and thallium imaging: Comparison of sensitivity and specificity. *Am. J. Cardiol.* 43:432.

Friedman, M. L.; and Cantor, R. E. 1979. Reliability of gated heart scintigrams for detection of left ventricular aneurysm. *J. Nucl. Med.* 20:720–23.

Frischknecht, J.; Steele, P.; Kirch, D., et al. 1979. Effects of exercise on left ventricular ejection fraction in men with coronary artery disease. *Am. Heart J.* 97:494–98.

Froehlich, R. T.; Falsetti, H. L.; and Doty, B. 1980. Prospective study of surgery for left ventricular aneurysm. *Am. J. Cardiol.* 45:923–30.

Gibbons, R. J.; Lee, K. L.; Cobb, F., et al. 1981. Ejection fraction response to exercise in patients with chest pain and normal coronary arteriograms. *Circulation* 64:952–57.

Jengo, J. A.; Oren, V.; Conant, R., et al. 1979. Effects of maximal exercise stress on left ventricular function in patients with coronary artery disease using first pass radionuclide angiocardiography: A rapid, noninvasive technique for determining ejection fraction and segmental wall motion. *Circulation* 59:60–65.

Johnson, L. L.; McCarthy, D. M.; Sciacca, R. R., et al. 1979. Right ventricular ejection fraction during exercise in patients with coronary artery disease. *Circulation* 60:1284–91.

Kent, K. M.; Borer, J. S.; Green, M. V., et al. 1978. Effects of coronary artery bypass on global and regional left ventricular function during exercise. *N. Engl. J. Med.* 298:1434–39.

Kirshenbaum, H. E.; Okada, R. D.; and Kushner, F. G. 1979. The relation of global left ventricular function with exercise to thallium-201 exercise scintigrams. *Clin. Res.* 27:180.

Links, J. M.; Becker, L. C.; Shindledecker, J. G., et al. 1982. Measurement of absolute left ventricular volume from gated blood pool studies. *Circulation* 65:82-90.

Maddahi, J.; Berman, D. S.; Matsuoka, D. T., et al. 1979. A new technique for assessing right ventricular ejection fraction using multiple-gated equilibrium cardiac blood pool scintigraphy. *Circulation* 60:581-87.

Maddox, D. E.; Wynne, J.; Uren, R., et al. 1979. Regional ejection fraction: A quantitative radionuclide index of regional left ventricular performance. *Circulation* 59:1001-09.

Marshall, R. C.; Berger, H. J.; Costin, J. C., et al., 1977. Assessment of cardiac performance with quantitative radionuclide angiography: Sequential left ventricular ejection fraction, normalized left ventricular ejection rate, and regional wall motion. *Circulation* 56:820-29.

Marshall, R. C.; Berger, H. J.; Reduto, L. A., et al. 1978. Assessment of cardiac performance with quantitative radionuclide angiography: Effects of oral propranolol on global and regional left ventricular function in coronary artery disease. *Circulation* 58:808-14.

Marshall, R.; Wisenberg, G.; Schelbert, H., et al. 1979. Radionuclide evaluation of the effect of oral propranolol on left ventricular function during exercise in patients with coronary artery disease. Abstract, *Am. J. Cardiol.* 43:398.

Morrison, J.; Coromilas, J.; Munsey, D., et al. 1980. Correlation of radionuclide estimates of myocardial infarction size and release of creatinine kinase-MB in man. *Circulation* 62:277-87.

Okada, R. D.; Boucher, C. A.; Strauss, H. W., et al. 1980. Exercise radionuclide imaging approaches to coronary artery disease. *Am. J. Cardiol.* 46:1188-1204.

Poliner, L.; Dehmer, G.; Lewis, S., et al. 1979. Comparison of supine and upright left ventricular performance by radionuclide ventriculography during rest and exercise in normal subjects. Abstract, *Circulation* 60:235.

Port, S.; Cobb, F. R.; Coleman, E., et al. 1980. Effect of age on the response of the left ventricular ejection fraction to exercise. *N. Engl. J. Med.* 303:1133-37.

Ramanathan, R. B.; Bodenheimer, M. M.; Banka, V. S., et al. 1979. Severity of contraction abnormalities after acute myocardial infarction in man: Response to nitroglycerin. *Circulation* 60:1230-37.

Reduto, L. A.; Berger, H. J.; Cohen, L. S., et al. 1978. Sequential radionuclide assessment of left and right ventricular performance after acute transmural myocardial infarction. *Ann. Intern. Med.* 89:441-47.

Rerych, S. K.; Scholz, P. M.; Newman, G. E., et al. 1978. Cardiac function at rest and during exercise in normals and in patients with coronary heart disease: Evaluation by radionuclide angiocardiography. *Ann. Surg.* 187:449-62.

Rigo, P.; Alderson, P. O.; Robertson, R. M., et al. 1979. Measurement of aortic and mitral regurgitation by gated cardiac blood pool scans. *Circulation* 60:306-12.

Ritchie, J. L.; Sorensen, S. G.; Kennedy, J. W., et al. 1979. Radionuclide angiography: Non-invasive assessment of hemodynamic changes after administration of nitroglycerin. *Am. J. Cardiol.* 43:278-84.

Salel, A. F.; Berman, D. S.; DeNardo, G. L., et al. 1976. Radionuclide assessment of nitroglycerin influence on abnormal left ventricular segmental contraction in patients with coronary heart disease. *Circulation* 53:975-82.

Schelbert, H. R.; Henning, H.; Ashburn, W. L., et al. 1976. Serial measurements of left ventricular ejection fraction by radionuclide angiography early and late after myocardial infarction. *Am. J. Cardiol.* 38:407-15.

Schelbert, H. R.; Verba, J. W.; Johnson, A. D., et al. 1975. Nontraumatic determination of left ventricular ejection fraction by radionuclide angiography. *Circulation* 51:902-09.

Slutsky, R.; Curtis, G.; Batler, A., et al. 1979. Effect of sublingual nitroglycerin on left ventricular function at rest and during spontaneous angina pectoris: Assessments with a radionuclide approach. *Am. J. Cardiol.* 44:1365-70.

Slutsky, R.; Gordon, D.; Karliner, J., et al. 1979. Assessment of early ventricular systole by first pass radionuclide angiography: Useful method for detection of left ventricular dysfunction at rest in patients with coronary artery disease. *Am. J. Cardiol.* 44:459-65.

Slutsky, R.; Karliner, J.; Ricci, D., et al. 1979a. Left ventricular volumes by gated equilibrium radionuclide angiography: A new method. *Circulation* 60:556-64.

———. 1979b. Response of left ventricular volume to exercise in man assessed by radionuclide equilibrium angiography. *Circulation* 60:565-72.

Tobinick, E.; Schelbert, H. R.; Henning, H., et al. 1978. Right ventricular ejection fraction in patients with acute anterior and inferior myocardial infarction assessed by radionuclide angiography. *Circulation* 57:1078-84.

Van Dyke, D.; Anger, H. O.; Sullivan, R. W., et al. 1972. Cardiac evaluation from radioisotope dynamics. *J. Nucl. Med.* 13:585-92.

Verani, M. S.; Del Ventura, L.; and Meller, R. R. 1979. Radionuclide ventriculograms during dynamic and isometric exercise in coronary artery disease: Comparison with exercise thallium-201 scintigrams. *Clin. Res.* 27:211.

Vogel, R. A.; Kirch, D. L.; LeFree, M. T., et al. 1979. Gated blood pool tomography using the seven pinhole Anger camera technique. Abstract, *Circulation* 60 suppl. II:36.

Winzelberg, G. G.; Miller, S. W.; Okada, R. D. et al. 1980. Scintigraphic assessment of false left ventricular aneurysm. *Am. J. Roentgenol.* 135:569–74.

Wynne, J.; Sayres, M.; Maddox, D. E., et al. 1980. Regional left ventricular function in acute myocardial infarction: Evaluation with quantitative radionuclide ventriculography. *Am. J. Cardiol.* 45:203–08.

Zaret, B. L.; Strauss, H. W.; Hurley, P. J., et al. 1971. A non-invasive scintiphotographic method for detecting regional ventricular dysfunction in man. *N. Engl. J. Med.* 284:1165–70.

8 Valvular Heart Disease

Jeffrey S. Borer, M.D.
Stephen L. Bacharach, Ph.D.
Michael V. Green, M.S.

Cardiology Division
Department of Medicine
New York Hospital—Cornell Medical Center
New York, New York

Division of Nuclear Medicine
Clinical Center
National Institutes of Health
Bethesda, Maryland

The patient with valvular regurgitation presents the physician with a particularly difficult management problem. Clinical assessment based on history, physical examination, and electrocardiography provides relatively limited insight into the functional state of the myocardium. However, until recently, the lack of easily applied and objective indicators of left ventricular performance has precluded the periodic assessment of myocardial function necessary for appropriate therapeutic decisions. As a result, symptomatic complaints have generally provided the criteria for timing valve replacement.

Recent prospective studies in patients with aortic regurgitation indicate that when the presence of congestive symptoms or marked exercise intolerance is used as the criterion for valve replacement, long-term postoperative results are poor (Henry, Bonow, Borer, et al., 1980; Henry, Bonow, Rosing, et al., 1980). In Henry and coworkers' assessment, five-year postoperative survival was only 60% and almost invariably the gradual development of severe left ventricular failure was the cause of late postoperative death. Prosthetic valve-related problems, such as paraprosthetic regurgitation, thromboembolic phenomena, and prosthesis orifice obstruction, were apparently not of importance in late postoperative mortality. In the patient with mitral regurgitation, the clinical course after development of symptoms appears to be somewhat more benign, but here as well the development of severe left ventricular dysfunction may be associated only with moderately severe symptoms.

As in the patient with aortic regurgitation, severe preoperative left ventricular dysfunction with mitral regurgitation is associated with depressed postoperative ventricular performance, most likely accounting for the residual symptomatic debility (Schuler, Peterson, et al., 1979). Moreover, in this patient the development of pulmonary hypertension often results in right ventricular dysfunction, the prognostic significance of which is only now being assessed (Hochreiter, Borer, et al., 1982).

The above-noted findings emphasized the inadequacy of symptom-based surgical criteria, and current valve-replacement procedures are not without short- and long-term risks. Perioperative mortality is approximately 5% for aortic valve replacement and 8% for mitral valve replacement, and intraoperative myocardial preservation techniques are not sufficient to preclude some degree of myocardial damage. Lifetime anticoagulation is necessary, with its attendant risk of hemorrhagic events, and even in patients with chronic anticoagulation, thromboembolic events occur with definable frequency. Paravalvular leakage can occur, with associated hemodynamic problems, and valve-related hemolysis is occasionally sufficient to require chronic transfusion therapy. The mechanical function of previously available valvular prostheses has been definably limited, and the effective life of currently available prostheses is as yet unknown. Thus, despite the obvious desirability of not withholding valve replacement until the development of clinical debility, the undesirable risks of premature valve replacement before the development of life-limiting left ventricular dysfunction must also be considered. As a result, many investigators have sought easily measured indices of left ventricular function that would be sufficiently predictive of clinical course to serve as a more rational basis for the surgical selection of asymptomatic patients.

AORTIC REGURGITATION

Studies of Henry, Bonow, Borer, et al. (1980) and Henry, Bonow, Rosing, et al. (1980) provided an important advance in the search for such objective criteria. These investigators employed echocardiography at rest to define preoperative left ventricular physical and function dimensions predictive of particularly poor long-term postoperative results for symptomatic patients. In addition, predictors of the imminent development of symptoms for a small, potentially high-risk group of asymptomatic patients who might otherwise benefit from surgery were also worked out. These landmark studies established the benefits of left ventricular function analysis in the determination of prognosis and operability for patients with aortic regurgitation.

However, in many patients with common forms of heart disease, abnormalities in left ventricular function only become apparent with myocardial stress, such as that associated with physical exercise. The development of radionuclide cineangiography, permitting the noninvasive assessment of left ventricular function both at rest and during maximal exercise, has provided a potential tool, better suited for refining the prognostic criteria based only on echocardiography performed at rest (Bacharach, Green, et al., 1977; Borer, Bacharach, et al., 1977, 1978a, 1978b, 1978c; Borer, Gottdiener, et al., 1979; Borer, Kent, et al., 1979; Borer, Rosing, et al., 1979).

At present, insufficient long-term data are available to permit accurate evaluation of the prognostic significance of exercise radionuclide cineangiography for patients with aortic regurgitation. However, studies to date indicate the sensitivity of the method for detection of left ventricular dysfunction in asymptomatic patients (Borer, Bacharach, et al., 1978b) and in predicting postoperative left ventricular function for symptomatic patients studied before valve replacement (Borer, Rosing, et al., 1979). The latter results suggest the potential utility of the method as a prognostic tool.

The earliest radionuclide cineangiographic assessment of patients with aortic regurgitation involved 43 patients, of whom 21 were symptomatic and 22 symptom-free. This study indicated the sensitivity of the method as performed during exercise for the detection of left ventricular dysfunction even in asymptomatic patients. It further documented the lack of distinction between symptomatic and asymptomatic patients when objective assessment of left ventricular function is performed (Borer, Bacharach, et al., 1978b).

All 43 patients manifested isolated aortic regurgitation, with ⩽10 mm Hg transvalvular pressure gradient and coronary arteries free of obstructions exceeding 30% of luminal diameter by coronary arteriography. Thirty normal subjects aged 10 to 63 years, free of symptoms and any abnormal physical, echocardiographic, or exercise electrocardiographic findings, were studied for purposes of comparison. The normal subjects were studied at three levels of exercise, so that the ejection fraction responses of patients, who often develop exercise-limiting fatigue or dyspnea at relatively low heart rates, could be compared with those of normal subjects at similar heart rates.

Ejection fractions in the normal subjects averaged 57% during rest and rose to 65% during mild exercise (heart rates 90/min to 105/min). At moderate exercise (heart rates 106/min to 120/min) this figure rose to 69%, and at maximal exercise (heart rate 121/min to 195/min; average 155/min) to 71%. Thus, normal subjects manifested their greatest increment in left ventricular ejection fraction on mild exercise. Subsequent increases in exercise intensity were associated with relatively small additions to the ejection fraction. In comparison, 21 symptomatic patients with aortic regurgitation manifested an average ejection fraction of 47% at rest, significantly below normal, although in 14 cases individual values were within the normal range (Figures 8-1 and 8-2). During maximal exercise, heart rates ranged from 99/min to 150/min (average 127/min), while the average injection fraction fell to 38%, remaining within normal limits for only one of the 21 patients and falling from previous resting values in 20 of the 21. Ejection fraction in 22 asymptomatic patients averaged 62% at rest, but fell to 57% during exercise, with heart rates ranging from 102/min to 171/min (average 134/min), a significantly ($p < .001$) subnormal value. While 21 of the 22 asymptomatic patients manifested normal ejection fractions at rest, nine of 22 developed subnormal values during maximal exercise.

Exercise ejection fractions could not be predicted from rest values and often were lower in asymptomatic patients than values recorded during exercise in symptomatic operative candidates. In addition, asymptomatic and symptomatic patients were not separable on the basis of echocardiographic left ventricular transverse dimension in diastole (a measure of left ventricular dilatation and, hence, of preload), peak systolic arterial pressure during exercise, left ventricular end-diastolic pressure at rest, or Romhilt-Estes ECG score for left ventricular hypertrophy. Moreover, the left ventricular ejection fraction correlated poorly, if at all, with these indicators of ventricular loading and size. Significant change in left ventricular end-diastolic volume was not associated with exercise in normal subjects, but an average 6% diminution occurred during exercise with aortic regurgitation. Moreover, the end-diastolic volume changes occurring during exercise were equivalent in the 14 patients with normal exercise

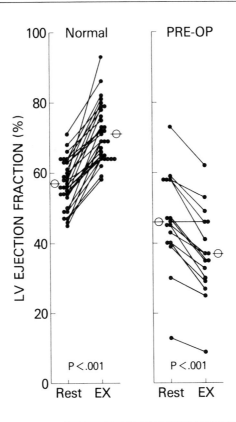

Figure 8-1 Effect of exercise on left ventricular ejection fraction in normal subjects and in symptomatic patients with aortic regurgitation. Note that most such patients manifest diminished left ventricular ejection fraction during exercise as compared with resting values, and most manifest absolute ejection fractions during exercise that are lower than the lowest value in any normal subject. EX, exercise; **PRE-OP**, before aortic valve replacement; **LV**, left ventricle. (Reproduced, in modified form, from Borer, J. S.; Rosing, D. R.; Kent, K. M., et al. 1979. *Am. J. Cardiol.* 44:1297–1305.)

ejection fractions and in the 29 patients with subnormal ejection fractions (Figure 8-3) (Borer, Bacharach, et al., 1978b).

Sixteen of the 21 symptomatic patients underwent aortic valve replacement and all returned six months after operation for cardiac catheterization and radionuclide cineangiography (Borer, Rosing, et al., 1979). Transprosthetic gradients varied between 0 mm Hg and 15 mm Hg and were ≥ 10 mm Hg in only five of 16 patients. Thus, ejection fractions were unlikely to be significantly affected by prosthesis-related abnormal-

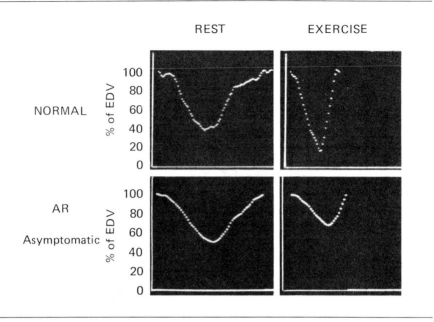

Figure 8-2 Time-activity curves obtained at rest and during maximum exercise in a normal subject and in a patient with aortic regurgitation who was totally asymptomatic. Approximately two-thirds of our totally asymptomatic patients with hemodynamically severe aortic regurgitation manifested a diminution in ejection fraction to subnormal levels during exercise, as exemplified by the results in this patient. **AR**, aortic regurgitation; **EDV**, end-diastolic volume. [Reproduced from *Cardiology update: Reviews for physicians*, 1979 (Elliot Rappaport, editor-in-chief). New York: Elsevier-North Holland, pp. 99–112.]

ities in left ventricular outflow impedance. Moreover, the average postsurgical left ventricular end-diastolic pressure fell to 11 mm Hg as compared with 18 mm Hg before operation ($p < .01$), while average echocardiographic end-diastolic dimension fell from 77 mm to 56 mm ($p < .001$). In 12 of 16 patients, the latter were within normal limits after operation. It is therefore concluded that abnormally elevated preload is not likely to be an important factor in causing ejection fraction abnormalities.

When assessed at rest, ejection fractions returned to normal after surgery, averaging 58% as compared with preoperative values of 46%. This indicates reversibility of at least part of preoperative myocardial dysfunction. Use of radionuclide cineangiography to aid in decisions regarding the timing of operation is based on the assumption that preoperative indices of left ventricular function are likely to predict postoperative functional deficits and that presence of the latter presumably indicates proclivity toward clinical debility. Therefore, the return of resting ejection fractions

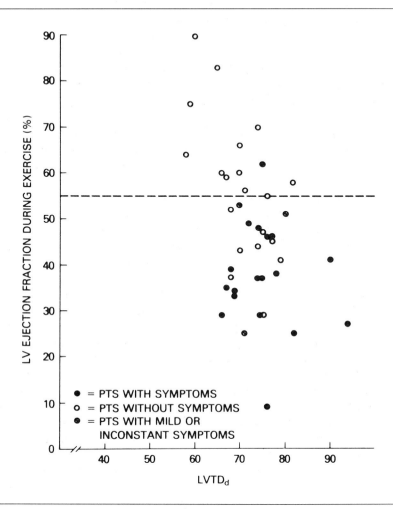

Figure 8-3 Relation between left ventricular ejection fraction during exercise and left ventricular end-diastolic volume as represented by echocardiographic left ventricular transverse dimension in diastole (LVTDd). (Reproduced from Borer, J. S.; Bacharach, S. L.; Green, M. V., et al. 1978. *Am. J. Cardiol.* 42:351-57.)

to normal after operation could be construed as indicating that preoperative radionuclide cineangiography is not likely to be predictive of long-term postoperative results. However, results of ejection fraction assessment during exercise indicate that, in fact, the preoperative functional lesion had not been totally mitigated by operation, emphasizing the potential value of exercise studies in patients with aortic regurgitation. The postsurgical ejection fraction during exercise averaged 52%, a significant increase compared with a preoperative value of 36% but significantly below the normal average of 71% and less than the lower limit of normal range, namely 55% (Figure 8-4). Thus, presurgical demonstration of subnormal exercise left ventricular function predicted the persistence of myocardial dysfunction after operation, even in the absence of postoperative abnormal left ventricular loading conditions. Moreover, in individual patients, the absolute value of the preoperative ejection fraction can reliably predict the likelihood of return to normal left ventricular function after operation. Thus, patients manifesting ejection fractions less than 40% during exercise before operation are highly unlikely to develop normal left ventricular function after valve replacement, irrespective of presurgical rest values.

While intraoperative myocardial injury could account for some of the functional impairment noted after surgery, it seems unlikely that this represents an important factor, since symptomatic patients undergoing aortic valve replacement for aortic stenosis generally manifest normal ejection fractions during exercise after valve replacement (Borer, Bacharach, et al., 1978c).

Analysis of exercise tolerance data in a larger group of patients before and after valve replacement suggests that conclusions regarding reversibility of preoperative systolic dysfunction can be modified to some extent by reference to preoperative exercise capacity (Bonow, Borer, et al., 1980). Thus, of 45 symptomatic patients, 27 manifested moderate exercise intolerance during treadmill testing before operation. The combination of subnormal resting systolic function and poor exercise tolerance before operation was particularly ominous. Within three years of operation, nine of 17 such patients died, almost always from late postoperative development of congestive heart failure, while no deaths occurred in a group of 15 patients with subnormal systolic function but normal treadmill results. Postoperative exercise ejection fraction, moreover, was significantly lower in patients with poor preoperative exercise tolerance than in those with more normal exercise capacity. The prognostic importance of these results is as yet unclear because of the paucity of preoperative radionuclide cineangiograms in the study group.

Preoperative analysis of echocardiographic end-systolic dimension during rest can be of value in identifying patients at particularly high risk after operation (Henry, Bonow, Borer, et al., 1980; Henry, Bonow, Rosing, et al., 1980). Recent results suggest that when patients with aortic regurgitation are segregated according to end-systolic dimension, subdivision within each group can be effected by the radionuclide cineangiographic assessment of left ventricular ejection fraction during exercise (Henry, Borer, et al., 1979). Thus, in our study, while virtually all patients in the echocardiographically defined high-risk group (end-systolic dimension ≥ 55 mm) manifested reduction in ejection fraction to subnormal values, the degree of exercise-induced dysfunction was variable and did

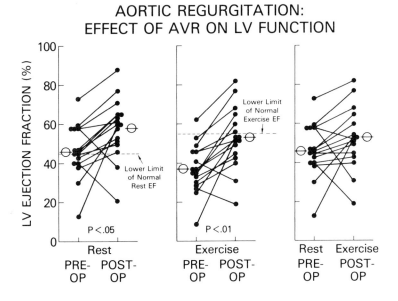

Figure 8-4 Effects of aortic valve replacement on left ventricular ejection fraction at rest and during exercise. **AVR**, aortic valve replacement. (Reproduced from Borer, J. S.; Rosing, D. R.; Kent, K. M., et al. 1979. *Am. J. Cardiol.* 44: 1297–1305.)

not correlate with abnormalities in the echocardiographic dimension. Among symptomatic patients with end-systolic dimensions of 45–54 mm and whose prognosis is generally good after operation (15% mortality within five years), exercise ejection fractions varied from normal to markedly subnormal. Such findings strongly suggest that assessment of prognosis, already possible to some extent on the basis of resting echocardiographic findings, can be further refined by reference to left ventricular function during exercise. Most recently, preliminary data from our laboratory have further supported this conclusion. Among 25 patients followed with noninvasive testing at yearly intervals, it was found that a fall in ejection fraction during exercise in year 1 was associated with a subsequent increase in echocardiographic end-systolic dimension in year 2, while the absence of a fall in ejection fraction during exercise in year 1 predicted the absence of change in end-systolic dimension in year 2. In fact, for patients with ejection fraction fall during exercise of greater than or equal to 5%, the average increase in end-systolic dimension during the ensuing year was 4.1 mm, a rather sizeable change (Hochreiter, Niles, et al., 1983).

In the consideration of the natural history of patients with aortic regurgitation, depression of left ventricular function during stress represents a mid-point between normal function and left ventricular dysfunction at rest. Extrapolation of current results for use in determining prognosis is not yet possible. The relationship of decreased exercise ejection fraction to long-term prognosis is as yet unknown. However, an assessment of ejection fraction during exercise may permit selection of patients for operation, after ventricular function has deteriorated sufficiently to justify the risk of operation but before myocardial damage has progressed to the point where postoperative prognosis is jeopardized. Further studies are required to determine the appropriate role of exercise radionuclide cineangiography in the selection of asymptomatic patients for valve replacement.

Because of the usefulness of myocardial perfusion scintigraphy with ^{201}Tl in the evaluation of patients with coronary artery disease, early attempts were made to employ myocardial perfusion scintigraphy in the evaluation of patients with valvular heart disease. As yet, no information of practical importance has emerged from such studies. In the early work of Bailey, Come, et al. (1977), myocardial perfusion scintigraphy was employed in the study of patients with aortic stenosis. All of the studies indicated that left ventricular wall thinning, suggestive of subendocardial ischemia, was detectable after exercise before aortic valve replacement, and often was absent after exercise following aortic valve replacement. Thus, it was suggested that myocardial perfusion scintigraphy might be of value in assessing the effectiveness of aortic valve replacement in such patients. However, no quantitation of the functional benefits of aortic valve replacement is possible with the myocardial perfusion scintigraphic technique. Moreover, focal perfusion defects, suggestive of the presence of large-vessel coronary artery stenoses, were noted in many patients who had no angiographic evidence of coronary artery stenosis, and in patients who had minor wall abnormalities of the coronary arteries. Thus, myocardial perfusion scintigraphy was found to be inaccurate in the identification of patients suffering from the combination of coronary artery occlusive disease and aortic valvular stenosis.

MITRAL REGURGITATION

Considerably less information is available regarding the value of radionuclide angiography for patients with mitral regurgitation.

Preliminary data were published in 1979 for a group of 20 symptomatic patients with isolated, hemodynamically severe mitral regurgitation (Borer, Gottdiener, et al., 1979). Of these, the left ventricular ejection fraction was normal in 18, but normal during exercise in only 10. The left ventricular ejection fraction was not related to symptoms; the average ejection fraction was 52% at rest and 56% during exercise for patients in New York Heart Association Functional Class II, 54% at rest and 54% during exercise in Functional Class III. Moreover, the ejection fraction at rest and during exercise did not correlate with either right ventricular loading conditions during exercise (right atrial or right ventricular pressures) or with left ventricular loading conditions during exercise (left atrial and left ventricular pressures and left ventricular volume). While these results provide only preliminary insight into the hemodynamic and myocardial function interrelationships that affect clinical outcome for patients with mitral regurgitation, they suggest that the ejection fraction can provide information regarding myocardial function status that is relatively independent of conventionally determined hemodynamic parameters. More recent data from our laboratory have suggested that, while left ventricular function may provide clinically useful information, assessment of right ventricular ejection fraction can be of particular value. We have found that, during exercise, right ventricular ejection fraction, but not left ventricular ejection fraction, is directly correlated with exercise tolerance. Right ventricular ejection fraction is inversely correlated with pulmonary artery pressure, a known prognostic index in patients with mitral regurgitation, and, together with left ventricular ejection fraction, can predict the likelihood of ventricular tachycardia in these patients (Hochreiter, Borer, et al., 1982). Further information regarding the importance of assessment of both left and right ventricular function awaits results of pre- and postoperative studies presently under way.

However, the subgroup of patients with mitral valve prolapse has been more extensively studied (Gottdiener, Borer, et al., 1981). Patients of greatest interest in this group are those with minimal mitral regurgitation because they often manifest chest discomfort indistinguishable from typical anginal pain. In a study of 39 such patients with chest pain and/or severe arrhythmias but without occlusive coronary artery disease, 36 manifested normal radionuclide cineangiographic results during exercise, although many of these developed abnormal ST segment responses during exercise electrocardiography. Thus, radionuclide cineangiography can be used to rule out coronary artery disease in more than 90% of patients with mitral valve prolapse and angina pain. In the remaining patients, who manifested ejection fraction abnormalities during exercise, the cause of dysfunction was unclear. However, recent evidence suggests the possibility of a more generalized cardiomyopathic process that can account for the exercise-induced dysfunction.

References

Bacharach, S. L.; Green, M. V.; Borer, J. S., et al. 1977. A real-time system for multi-image gated cardiac studies. *J. Nucl. Med.* 18:79–84.

Bailey, I. K.; Come, P. C.; Kelley, D. T., et al. 1977. Thallium-201 myocardial perfusion imaging in aortic valve stenosis. *Am. J. Cardiol.* 40:889–99.

Bonow, R. O.; Borer, J. S.; Rosing, D. R., et al. 1980. Preoperative exercise capacity in patients with aortic regurgitation as a predictor of postoperative left ventricular function and long-term prognosis. *Circulation* 62:1280–90.

Borer, J. S.; Bacharach, S. L.; Green, M. V., et al. 1977. Real-time radionuclide cineangiography in the non-invasive evaluation of global and regional left ventricular function at rest and during exercise in patients with coronary artery disease. *N. Engl. J. Med.* 296:839–44.

———. 1978a. Effect of nitroglycerin on exercise-induced abnormalities of left ventricular regional function and ejection fraction in coronary artery disease: Assessment by radionuclide cineangiography in symptomatic and asymptomatic patients. *Circulation* 57:314–20.

———. 1978b. Exercise-induced left ventricular dysfunction in symptomatic and asymptomatic patients with aortic regurgitation: Assessment by radionuclide cineangiography. *Am. J. Cardiol.* 42:351–57.

———. 1978c. Left ventricular function in aortic stenosis: Response to exercise and effects of operation. Abstract, *Am. J. Cardiol.* 41:382.

Borer, J. S.; Gottdiener, J. S.; Rosing, D. R., et al. 1979. Left ventricular function in mitral regurgitation: Determination during exercise. Abstract, *Circulation* 60 (suppl. II):38.

Borer, J. S.; Kent, K. M.; Bacharach, S. L., et al. 1979. Sensitivity, specificity and predictive accuracy of radionuclide cineangiography during exercise in patients with coronary artery disease: Comparison with exercise electrocardiography. *Circulation* 60:572–80.

Borer, J. S.; Rosing, D. R.; Kent, K. M., et al. 1979. Left ventricular function at rest and during exercise after aortic valve replacement in patients with aortic regurgitation. *Am. J. Cardiol.* 44:1297–1305.

Gottdiener, J. S.; Borer, J. S.; Bacharach, S. L., et al. 1981. Left ventricular function in mitral valve prolapse: Assessment with radionuclide cineangiography. *Am. J. Cardiol.* 47:7–13.

Henry, W. L.; Bonow, R. O.; Borer, J. S., et al. 1980. Observations on the optimum time for operative intervention for aortic regurgitation. I. Evaluation of the results of aortic valve replacement in symptomatic patients. *Circulation* 61:471–83.

Henry, W. L.; Bonow, R. O.; Rosing, D. R., et al. 1980. Observations on the optimum time for operative intervention for aortic regurgitation. II. Serial echocardiographic evaluation of asymptomatic patients. *Circulation* 61:484–92.

Henry, W. L.; Borer, J. S.; Bonow, R. O., et al. 1979. Functional adaptations of the left ventricle to chronic aortic regurgitation. Abstract, *Am. J. Cardiol.* 43:412.

Hochreiter, C.; Borer, J. S.; Devereux, R., et al. 1982. Right ventricular function in mitral regurgitation: Predictive value clinically? Abstract, *Circulation* 66 (suppl. II):II–355.

Hochreiter, C.; Niles, N.; Borer, J. S., et al. 1983. Increasing left ventricular systolic dimension in aortic regurgitation predicted by previous exercise left ventricular function. Abstract, *Clin. Res.* 31:664A.

Schuler, G.; Peterson, K. L.; Johnson, A., et al. 1979. Temporal response of left ventricular performance to mitral valve surgery. *Circulation* 59:1218–31.

9 Cardiomyopathies

Maurice N. Druck, M.D.

Staff Cardiologist
Director of Non-Invasive Cardiology
    and Nuclear Cardiology Laboratory
Toronto Western Hospital
Toronto, Ontario, Canada

The cardiomyopathies include a group of pathologic entities that primarily affect heart muscle and specifically exclude ischemic, hypertensive, valvular, congenital, and pericardial disease. Various classifications have been proposed. The first divides the cardiomyopathies into primary and secondary forms. Primary cardiomyopathies include those entities in which the underlying process involves only the myocardium; the cause is unknown. Secondary cardiomyopathies are those in which the myocardial disease is secondary to a systemic process such as sarcoidosis. A second classification is etiological and is based on identification of a specific cause (Table 9-1). In a large number of cases the etiology cannot be identified and the term idiopathic is applied.

A third and more useful classification is functional. It is based on three categories:

1. Congestive or dilated cardiomyopathy, with left ventricular dilatation and poor systolic function.

2. Restrictive cardiomyopathy, with decreased left ventricular compliance, small or normal-sized left ventricle, and normal systolic function.

3. Hypertrophic cardiomyopathy, characterized by a small or normal left ventricle, vigorous systolic function, and asymmetrical septal hypertrophy.

Radionuclide imaging techniques can be used to differentiate between the various categories, to follow the course of ventricular function, and to evaluate the response to therapeutic interventions. Gated cardiac blood pool imaging can be used to determine ventricular size, ventricular ejection fraction, configuration, wall motion, septal size and shape. With this information, cardiomyopathies can be functionally classified as congestive, restrictive, or hypertrophic. Since other heart diseases can simulate primary myocardial disease, it is often useful to image the heart with thallium-201. Patchy myocardial uptake implies cardiomyopathy and can usually be distinguished from regional perfusion abnormalities. In this way it is possible to distinguish primary congestive from ischemic congestive cardiomyopathy.

CONGESTIVE CARDIOMYOPATHY

Idiopathic congestive cardiomyopathy is the most common form and is characterized by biventricular failure, ventricular dilatation with excessive hypertrophy, and normal coronary arteries. Pathologically, a diffuse interstitial fibrosis or focal fibrosis can be seen (Roberts and Ferrans, 1975). The gated blood pool angiogram of patients with congestive cardiomyopathy presents typical findings (Figure 9-1), with both ventricles dilated and with a global decrease in wall motion. The left ventricle is usually more involved than the right, exhibiting an ejection fraction of more than

Table 9-1 Secondary Cardiomyopathy

A. Neuromuscular disease
   1. Friedreich's ataxia
   2. Myotonic muscular dystrophy
   3. Duchenne muscular dystrophy
   4. Facioscapulohumeral muscular dystrophy
   5. Limb-girdle muscular dystrophy

B. Connective tissue disease
   1. Scleroderma
   2. Dermatomyositis
   3. Rheumatoid heart disease
   4. Rheumatic myocardial disease
   5. Disseminated lupus erythematosus
   6. Ankylosing spondylitis

C. Neoplastic heart disease: primary and metastatic neoplasm, lymphoma, leukemia

D. Metabolic disease
   1. Thyrotoxicosis
   2. Hemochromatosis
   3. Myxedema
   4. Glycogen storage disease (Pompe's disease)
   5. Infiltrative diseases, e.g., Refsum's disease, mucopolysaccharidosis, Hunter's syndrome, Hurler's syndrome, the lipidoses
   6. Pheochromocytoma
   7. Acromegaly
   8. Diabetes mellitus

E. Nutritional disease
   1. Beriberi
   2. Kwashiorkor

F. Myocarditis
   1. Viral: Coxsackie B, Coxsackie A, influenza virus, infectious mononucleosis, poliovirus, mumps, chickenpox, smallpox, vaccinia, psittacosis, lymphogranuloma venereum, herpes simplex, cytomegalovirus, infectious hepatitis, German measles, rabies, yellow fever
   2. Parasitic: trichinosis
   3. Protozoal: trypanosomiasis (Cruz-Chagas disease), syphilis, toxoplasmosis, amebiasis, Borrelia recurrentis
   4. Bacterial: bacterial endocarditis, septicemia, diphtheria
   5. Unknown or allergic: drug reaction (e.g., penicillin) Loeffler's parietal endocarditis, serum sickness

G. Granulomatous cardiomyopathy: sarcoidosis

H. Amyloidosis
   1. Primary
      a. Senile
      b. Familial
      c. Nonfamilial
   2. Secondary

I. Posttraumatic cardiomyopathy: following penetrating or nonpenetrating trauma or surgical procedures

J. Toxic cardiomyopathy
   1. Uremia
   2. Alcoholism
   3. Carbon monoxide poisoning
   4. Phenothiazine and related drugs
   5. Cobalt
   6. Physical agents: radiation therapy, heatstroke, lightning
   7. Other drugs and chemical agents: adriamycin

Note: Reproduced, by permission of J. B. Lippincott/Harper & Row, from Fowler, N.O. 1976. *Cardiac diagnosis and treatment*. Hagerstown, MD: Harper & Row.

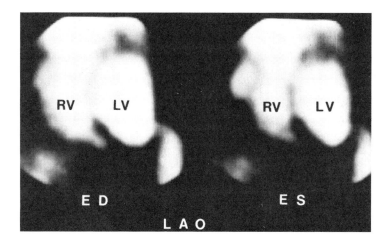

Figure 9-1 End-diastolic and end-systolic frames from the left anterior oblique (LAO) study of a patient with congestive cardiomyopathy. Note the dilated left ventricle with concentrically reduced wall motion. The right ventricle is contracting normally.

30%. Atria and the pulmonary arteries are often easily visualized, secondary to left ventricular failure. Wall motion is usually concentrically decreased, but the apical segment is often akinetic or dyskinetic. Although patients with repeated myocardial infarction can resemble those with congestive cardiomyopathy by gated nuclear angiogram, in ischemic heart disease the anterobasal and posterobasal segments often move normally, while in congestive cardiomyopathy this is not seen.

Thallium-201 imaging can also help to distinguish congestive from ischemic cardiomyopathy. With congestive cardiomyopathy, ^{201}Tl imaging usually demonstrates ventricular dilatation and a normal or diffuse reduction in myocardial uptake (Figure 9-2). Bulkley, Hutchins, et al. (1977) have indicated, using ^{201}Tl scintigraphy, that at least 40% of the myocardium in patients with ischemic cardiomyopathy will show a defect at rest. Figure 9-2 shows ^{201}Tl images in a patient with congestive cardiomyopathy; Figure 9-3, normal exercise and 3-hour ^{201}Tl images; and Figure 9-4, exercise and 3-hour ^{201}Tl images in a patient with ischemic cardiomyopathy.

Serial gated blood pool scanning can also be used to follow results of therapy. We have found it useful to assess patients with congestive cardiomyopathy before initiation of vasodilator therapy. If both rest and exercise gated nuclear angiograms are performed before and after medication, patients can be classified either as "responders" or "nonresponders."

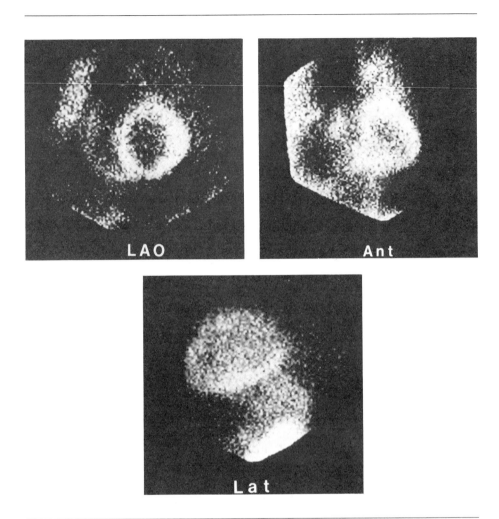

Figure 9-2 Exercise ^{201}Tl images in a patient with congestive cardiomyopathy showing an enlarged left ventricle, patchy defects, and increased lung uptake of thallium-201 seen best in the LAO view.

Responders may ultimately be placed on chronic vasodilator therapy, with good results. Nonresponders may not respond because left ventricular dysfunction may be past the point of no return, even with vasodilator therapy.

Rest and exercise gated nuclear angiography can be used as a guide in following patients receiving doxorubicin treatment for malignant disease (Alexander, Dainiak, et al., 1979; Druck, Bar-Shlomo, et al., 1981). It can reliably be used to predict and follow the course of doxorubicin cardiomyopathy, and with this technique, patients may be allowed

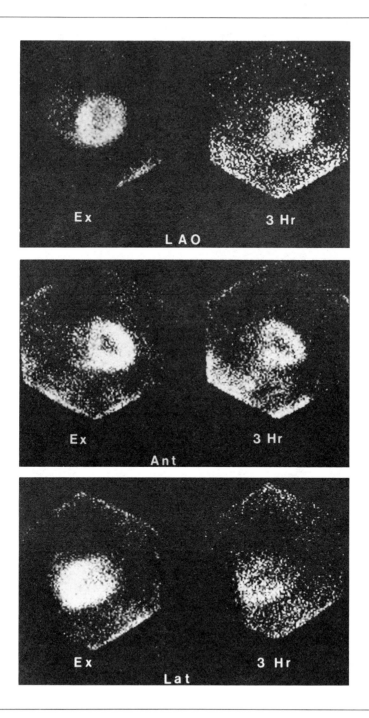

Figure 9-3 Normal exercise and 3-hour ^{201}Tl images.

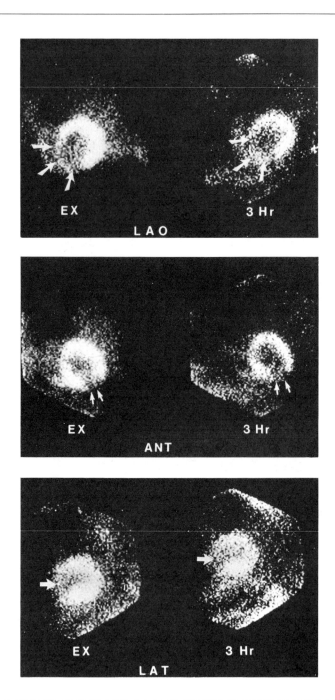

Figure 9-4 Exercise and 3-hour ^{201}Tl imaging in a patient with "ischemic cardio-myopathy" showing a segmental defect (arrows) persisting in the wash-in study, suggesting previous infarction.

.o receive high total cumulative doses without significant heart failure. Other patients, who might otherwise develop cardiomyopathic changes at doses far less than 550 mg/m^2, may be protected by early discontinuation of the drug. Our current approach to patients receiving doxorubicin, using gated nuclear angiography, is detailed in Figure 9-5.

RESTRICTIVE CARDIOMYOPATHY

Restrictive cardiomyopathy is the least common form seen in North America. It presents as a normal or small heart with signs of left and/or right ventricular failure. The markedly diminished ventricular compliance is caused by infiltration or fibrosis of the myocardium. Typical gated

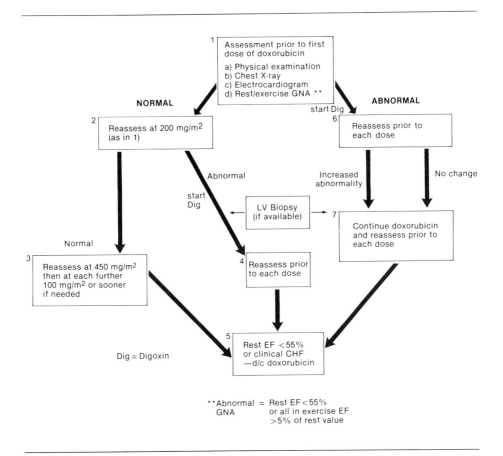

Figure 9-5 Our approach to patients receiving doxorubicin chemotherapy for malignant disease.

nuclear angiography findings in restrictive cardiomyopathy include normal or reduced end-diastolic ventricular size, usually associated with normal systolic function. Two subdivisions of restrictive cardiomyopathy are infiltrative cardiomyopathy, in which normal or slightly decreased ventricular cavities are seen with normal or hypertrophied walls; and obliterative cardiomyopathy, in which the left and/or right ventricular cavity is partially obliterated. Causes of the first include scleroderma, amyloidosis, hemochromatosis, glycogen storage disease, metastatic carcinoma, lymphoma, and leukemia. Causes of the second include endocardial fibrosis and endomyocardial fibrosis.

Gated nuclear angiography can help distinguish restrictive from congestive cardiomyopathy. In the latter the ventricular chambers are diffusely enlarged (Figure 9-1), but in the restrictive form, ventricular size is small or normal. Gated nuclear angiograms can also help distinguish restrictive cardiomyopathy from constrictive pericarditis. In constrictive pericarditis both ventricles usually have normal systolic function, whereas in restrictive cardiomyopathy there is usually a mild biventricular dysfunction. In obliterative disease an unusual configuration of the left ventricle is seen.

Thallium-201 imaging can also be useful in restrictive cardiomyopathy when neoplastic involvement of the myocardium is considered. Multiple large defects are seen, which helps to distinguish left ventricular dysfunction from that caused by other cardiac disease or toxic agents.

HYPERTROPHIC CARDIOMYOPATHY

Hypertrophic cardiomyopathy is a disease of unknown etiology characterized by asymmetric ventricular hypertrophy in which the septum is disproportionately thickened, especially with respect to the posterior left ventricular wall. Obstruction of left ventricular outflow may be present and is caused by a combination of septal hypertrophy and abnormal systolic movement of the anterior mitral valve leaflet (Braunwald, Morrow, et al., 1960; Wigle, Adelman, et al. 1971). Although echocardiography can be used to diagnose both of these, they can also relate to other entities and are not specific for hypertrophic cardiomyopathy (Shah, Gramiak, et al., 1969; Larter, Allen, et al., 1976; Crawford, Groves, et al., 1978; Marion, Gottdiener, et al., 1978; Mintz, Kitler, et al., 1978).

Nuclear techniques, including both gated nuclear angiography and ^{201}Tl imaging, can be helpful in the diagnosis of hypertrophic cardiomyopathy. Interventricular septal configuration can be detailed in the 40° to 50° left anterior oblique view of the gated nuclear angiogram. The normal septum (Figure 9-6) is curved and concave towards the left ventricle. In hypertrophic cardiomyopathy the interventricular septum is characteristically abnormal and can be visualized. Pohost and coworkers (1977) have demonstrated disproportionate upper septal thickening in 50% of patients with hypertrophic cardiomyopathy, and loss of normal

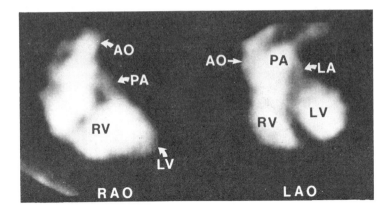

Figure 9-6 End-diastolic frames in right anterior and left anterior oblique views from a normal patient study. Note septal configuration with concavity towards the left ventricle.

septal concavity towards the left ventricle in 71% of patients (Figure 9-7). The gated scan can show cavity obliteration, apex obliteration, or mid-ventricular obstruction in the anterior or 30° right anterior oblique view (Figure 9-8).

Thallium-201 can also be used. Bulkley and coworkers (1975) compared septal to posterior left ventricular wall thickness in 10 patients. In patients with hypertrophic cardiomyopathy the basal and mid-posterior walls were equal in thickness, while in those with nonobstructive cardiomyopathy the basal wall was thinner than the mid-posterior wall. Configuration of the interventricular septum on ungated ^{201}Tl imaging showed a triangular-shaped septum, with the inferoapical segment thicker than the basal portion. This is in contrast to the disproportionate upper septal thickening seen on gated nuclear angiography and mentioned previously. Thallium-201 images are not usually gated with the electrocardiographic signal, and each image is therefore a composite of both the systolic and diastolic phases. In systole the left ventricular cavity is almost completely obliterated and gives the impression that the apical septum is thicker. Gated ^{201}Tl scanning shows a configuration similar to that of the gated nuclear angiogram (Mews, Pohost, et al., 1978).

Patients with hypertrophic cardiomyopathy have been subdivided into three classes: nonobstructive, latent obstructive, and resting obstructive, as determined by both M-mode and two-dimensional echocardiography (Gilbert, Pollick, et al., 1980). These subdivisions have been shown to be important in the management of patients. Pollick, Bar-Shlomo, et al. (1980) have demonstrated that it is also possible to differentiate these

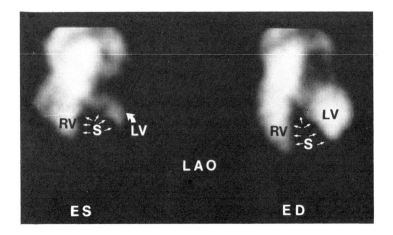

Figure 9-7 End-diastolic and end-systolic frames from the LAO study of a patient with hypertrophic cardiomyopathy. Note the massively thickened system with loss of normal concavity seen in Figure 9-6.

three classes with rest and exercise gated nuclear angiography. Patients with nonobstructive hypertrophic cardiomyopathy were found to have normal left ventricular ejection fractions both at rest and during exercise. Those with latent obstructive cardiomyopathy tended to have a high resting left ventricular ejection fraction that increased with exercise. Resting obstructive cardiomyopathy was also associated with a high resting ejection fraction, although as a group these patients tended to have an abnormal exercise response. It has been concluded, therefore, that significant differences in ventricular function at rest and during exercise can be demonstrated between the subdivisions of hypertrophic cardiomyopathy, and that the importance of functional hemodynamic classification in the management of these patients should be emphasized.

SUMMARY

Although the primary approach to the diagnosis of cardiomyopathy remains that of history, physical examination, electrocardiography, echocardiography, and chest X-ray, radionuclide techniques can provide useful information for the evaluation and management of patients with various forms of the disease. Gated nuclear angiography supplies information concerning ventricular ejection fraction, size, configuration, wall motion, and septal size and configuration; these data help determine the functional class of the cardiomyopathy. Thallium-201 imaging can be used to help differentiate congestive from ischemic cardiomyopathy and to detect

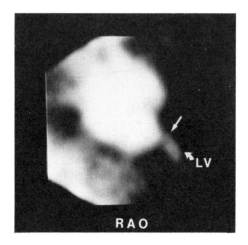

Figure 9-8 Right anterior oblique view of a patient with hypertrophic cardio-myopathy and mid-ventricular obstruction at the site indicated by the straight arrow.

septal abnormalities in hypertrophic cardiomyopathy. In addition, diseases that replace or displace myocardial cells (fibrosis, metastases) can also be detected by ^{201}Tl imaging. Finally, gated ^{201}Tl imaging can be useful for the detection of septal abnormalities in hypertrophic cardio-myopathy. In some instances the use of noninvasive techniques, including gated radionuclide angiography and/or ^{201}Tl imaging, may obviate the need for invasive methods, including cardiac catheterization and/or biopsy.

References

Alexander, J.; Dainiak, N.; Berger, H. J., et al. 1979. Serial assessment of doxorubicin cardiotoxicity with quantitative radionuclide angiocardio-graphy. *N. Engl. J. Med.* 300:278-83.

Braunwald, E.; Morrow, A. G.; Cornell, W. P., et al. 1960. Idiopathic hypertrophic subaortic stenosis: Clinical, hemodynamic, and angiographic manifestations. *Am. J. Med.* 29:924-45.

Bulkley, B. H.; Hutchins, G. M.; Bailey, I., et al. 1977. Thallium-201 imaging and gated cardiac blood pool scans in patients with ischemic and congestive cardiomyopathy: A clinical and pathologic study. *Circulation* 55: 753-60.

Bulkley, B. H.; Rouleau, J.; Strauss, H. W., et al. 1975. Idiopathic hypertrophic subaortic stenosis: Detection by thallium-201 myocardial perfusion imaging. *N. Engl. J. Med.* 293:1113-16.

Crawford, M. H.; Groves, B. M.; and Horwitz, L. D. 1978. Dynamic left ventricular outflow tract obstruction and systolic anterior motion of the mitral valve in the absence of asymmetric septal hypertrophy. *Am. J. Med.* 67:703-08.

Druck, M. N.; Bar-Schlomo, B. Z.; Gulenchyn, K. Y., et al. 1981. Radionuclide angiography and endomyocardial biopsy in the assessment of doxorubicin cardiotoxicity. Abstract, *Am. J. Cardiol.* 47:401.

Gilbert, B. W.; Pollick, C.; Adelman, A. G., et al. 1980. Hypertrophic cardiomyopathy: Subclassification by M mode echocardiography. *Am. J. Cardiol.* 45:861-72.

Larter, W. E.; Allen, H. D.; Sahn, D. J., et al. 1976. The asymmetrically hypertrophied septum: Further differentiation of its causes. *Circulation* 53:19-27.

Marion, B. J.; Gottdiener, J. S.; Roberts, W. C., et al. 1978. Left ventricular outflow tract obstruction due to systolic anterior motion of the anterior mitral valve leaflet in patients with concentric left ventricular hypertrophy. *Circulation* 57:527.

Mews, G. C.; Pohost, G. M.; Vignola, P. A., et al. 1978. Hypertrophic cardiomyopathy: Improved radionuclide detection by gated Tl-201 imaging. Abstract, *Circulation* 58 (suppl. II):II-236.

Mintz, G. S.; Kotler, M. N.; Segal, B. L., et al. 1978. Systolic anterior motion in the absence of asymmetric septal hypertrophy. *Circulation* 57: 256-63.

Pohost, G. M.; Vignola, P. A.; McKusick, K. E., et al. 1977. Hypertrophic cardiomyopathy: Evaluation by gated cardiac blood pool scanning. *Circulation* 55:92-99.

Pollick, C.; Bar-Shlomo, B.; McLaughlin, P., et al. 1980. Hypertrophic cardiomyopathy: Ventricular function studies by radionuclide angiography, Abstract, *Circulation* 62 (suppl. III):III-302.

Roberts, W. C.; and Ferrans, V. J. 1975. Pathologic anatomy of the cardiomyopathies: Idiopathic dilated and hypertrophic types, infiltrative types, and endomyocardial disease with and without eosinophilia. *Hum. Pathol.* 6:278-342.

Shah, P. M.; Gramiak, R.; and Kramer, D. H. 1969. Ultrasound localization of left ventricular obstruction in hypertrophic obstructive cardiomyopathy. *Circulation* 40:3-11.

Wigle, E. D.; Adelman, A. G.; and Silver, W. D. 1971. Pathophysiological considerations in muscular subaortic stenosis. In *Hypertrophic obstructive cardiomyopathy*. Ciba Foundation Study Group No. 37, edited by G. E. W. Wolstenholme, M. O'Connor, J. London, and A. Aronclife, London: Churchill-Livingstone.

10 Assessment of Congenital Heart Disease

Gary F. Gates, M.D.

Clinical Professor of Diagnostic Radiology
University of Oregon School of Medicine

Director of Nuclear Medicine
Good Samaritan Hospital and Medical Center
Portland, Oregon

During the past decade, a great variety of nuclear medicine tests have been developed for the evaluation of cardiac disease. However, because most tests are devised in response to the clinical needs of a specific patient population, pediatric and adult nuclear cardiographic examinations have developed as divergent branches of the specialty, often along parallel but separate lines.

Any nuclear cardiographic test performed in an adult can also be done in a child, although there are fewer times that myocardial infarct imaging or thallium scanning will be performed in a child than in an adult. However, 201-thallium perfusion imaging has been used to detect right ventricular hypertrophy (as in cyanotic heart disease) or the absence of an interventricular septum (as with a single ventricle). Myocardial ischemia can also be detected by ^{201}Tl in conditions such as anomalous left coronary artery, coarctation of the aorta, aortic valvular or subvalvular stenosis, neonatal asphyxia, and Kawasaki's disease.

Nuclear medicine examinations in children suspected of having heart disease are usually concerned with the detection and quantitation of cardiac shunts, evaluation of abnormalities of the great vessels, the discovery of anomalies of size or number of cardiac chambers, or the evaluation of postoperative effects of corrective cardiac surgery or of palliative systemic-to-pulmonic shunts. Three different sets of examinations can make these determinations: nuclear angiocardiography, left-to-right shunt quantitation, and right-to-left shunt quantitation. Although there is some overlap between the first two studies, the examinations are sufficiently distinct to warrant separate discussion.

NUCLEAR ANGIOCARDIOGRAPHY

Nuclear angiocardiography is similar to cardiac angiography done in a radiology department: a tracer agent (a radionuclide) is used to produce images of the route followed by blood as it flows through the heart and great vessels. However, nuclear techniques do not entail cardiac catheterization, use of iodinated contrast agents, heavy sedation, hospitalization, or high radiation exposures.

The radionuclide examination is performed by rapidly injecting ^{99m}Tc pertechnetate into either a basilic or external jugular vein. Before the injection, the child is placed before a scintillation camera, which is usually interfaced with a digital computer or a multiimage formating device that is capable of producing a rapid sequence of one-second images (Figure 10-1). Depending upon patient size, a parallel-hole, converging, or pinhole collimator may be used. The examination requires no particular patient preparation (except for mild sedation sometimes), and is concluded, from the patient's standpoint, about 30 to 60 seconds after radionuclide injection.

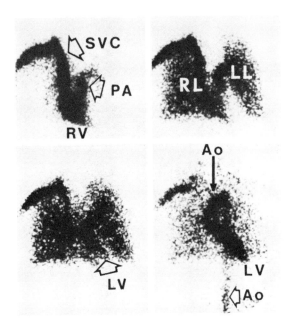

Figure 10-1 A series of one-second analog images obtained during a normal nuclear angiocardiogram show superior vena cava (**SVC**), right ventricle (**RV**), pulmonary artery (**PA**), right and left lungs (**RL, LL**), left ventricle (**LV**), plus ascending and descending aorta (**Ao**, upper and lower arrows, respectively).

There are many advantages to the use of a computer, including image processing and generation of time-activity curves from selected areas of interest such as cardiac chambers, lungs, and great vessels. The computer gives the option of recombining the many frames of raw data into desired images so that, for example, left and right sides of the heart can be superimposed and shown without displaying lung activity (Figure 10-2).

Interpretation of nuclear angiocardiograms is similar to the analysis of the corresponding radiographic studies. When evaluating the study of a patient suspected of having congenital heart disease, the observer must answer two basic questions: How many cardiac chambers can be identified and what is the time sequence of their visualization? What is the arrangement of the great vessels (i.e., aorta and pulmonary artery) and is there premature aortic visualization?

Analysis of nuclear images usually allows for easy visualization of both ventricles and the right atrial region, although it may be difficult to identify the left atrium as a separate structure. Cardiac valve location is

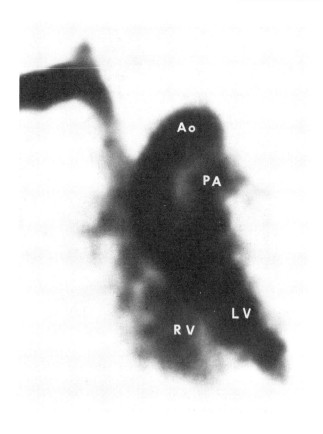

Figure 10-2 Computer-processed image showing a composite of total heart plus great vessels but excluding lungs.

usually inferred by watching sequential replays of the study, but of course the valves themselves are not seen directly. Visual inspection of nuclear angiocardiographic images allows the observer to identify a variety of congenital heart lesions (Jones and Anderson, 1975):

1. Left-to-right cardiac shunts. Continual visualization of the cardiac chambers with persistent lung imaging is a characteristic feature of these intracardiac shunts. Such shunting continually directs radionuclide-containing blood back into the right side of the heart, which in turn never empties in a normal manner. Excessive pulmonary artery flow and poor aortic flow may be evident in the apparent sizes of the vessels. Depending upon the location of the cardiac defect that is producing the shunt, the right atrium may or may not be as evi-

dent as the right ventricle. A later section will deal with specifics of shunt calculation.

2. Right-to-left shunts. Visualization of the aorta before one can image the pulmonary artery or lungs is a characteristic feature of this type of shunting. At times the right side of the heart may seem enlarged. A method of shunt quantitation will be discussed.

3. Patent ductus arteriosus. The observer sees the pulmonary artery persistently during aortic imaging without simultaneously visualizing the right heart. The left ventricle may be enlarged.

4. Transposition of the great vessels. The aorta is visualized directly after right heart visualization, but neither the pulmonary artery nor the left ventricle is seen.

5. Tetralogy of Fallot. In this anomaly there is premature filling of the aorta directly from the right ventricle, and visualization of the pulmonic outflow tract is poor.

6. Tricuspid atresia. The most striking observation in this disorder is the radionuclide flow from right to left atrium. Thereafter the observer sees the left ventricle and aorta. Later filling via a ventricular septal defect may show a small right ventricle.

7. Ebstein's anomaly. Prolonged tracer retention within its cavity will demonstrate a high right atrium. This situation is similar to that which may be seen in severe tricuspid insufficiency (Figure 10-3).

8. Congenital aortic or pulmonic stenosis. Depending upon the location of the stenotic lesion, the observer may see a supravalvular or subvalvular narrowing of the ejected column of radionuclide-containing blood. On occasion he or she may recognize poststenotic dilatation of the vessel.

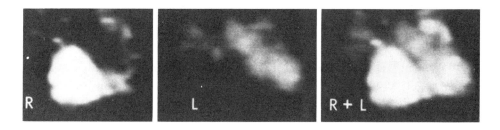

Figure 10-3 Tricuspid insufficiency following repair of ventricular septal defect. Separate right (R) and left (L) heart frames show large right atrial region, with its disproportionate size well shown on composite cardiac image (R + L).

LEFT-TO-RIGHT-SHUNT QUANTITATION

Quantitation of the left-to-right shunts requires the performance of a radionuclide angiocardiogram with computer analysis of the resultant data. Various areas of interest can be placed over the cardiac chambers and great vessels in order to show the presence of a shunt, but lung time-activity curves must be analyzed to quantitate its magnitude. The normal lung curve is composed of an initial rapid up-slope reaching a well-defined peak followed by a down-slope or washout component that theoretically would fall to baseline if it were not for the subsequent recirculation or "second pass" of radionuclide through the lungs. When a left-to-right shunt is present, the indicator recirculation curve will become abnormal, and the degree of abnormality will be proportional to the magnitude of shunting. The observed abnormality is based on the bypassing of the systemic circulation by the labeled blood which makes an early appearance in the pulmonary circulation. The magnitude of curve distortion is related to the size of the shunt and is the basis of shunt quantitation (Alazraki, Ashburn, et al., 1972).

The three methods of curve analysis used in quantitating left-to-right shunts are all based on the lung time-activity curves. Anderson, Jones, et al. (1974) have plotted lung counts derived from radionuclide angiocardiograms on semilogarithmic paper and extrapolated the initial descent of the first pass curve to a point equivalent to 1% of the peak height of the curve. This extrapolated line forms the division between two areas, Y and X, that roughly correspond to the first and second pass components of the pulmonary curve, respectively. The outer limits of the regions are formed by lines drawn perpendicular to the base line and passing through the peak of the first pass curve (for region Y) or perpendicular to the base line at the extrapolated 1% point of the down-slope curve to the intercept point on the actual lung curve (for area X). The ratio of the areas under the curves bounded by the X and Y limits is used to determine left-to-right shunting.

The C_2/C_1 technique (Alazraki, Ashburn, et al., 1972; Rosenthall and Mercer, 1973), an empirical method of curve analysis, is useful in shunt detection. The technique involves determination of the peak counts (C_1) of the lung curve and the time in the study at which C_1 occurs (T_1). The counts at a second point (C_2) on the curve are then determined by location of a second time point (T_2), which is the same interval from T_1 as the latter was from the appearance of tracer within the lungs. Normally the C_2/C_1 count ratio is about 0.3 to 0.35. Abnormal lung recirculation increases this ratio, which is really an index of shunting rather than an absolute measurement of the pulmonic:systemic flow ratio. However, this method is easy to perform and has good clinical utility in separating normals from abnormals.

In 1973, Maltz and Treves described a third method of curve analysis that makes use of the gamma variate function. This mathematical function dissects the pulmonary curve into its component parts: the first pass curve and the subsequent recirculation curve. The up-slope and initial portion of the down-slope of the pulmonary curve are unaffected by recirculation; a gamma variate function can be used to construct an isolated first pass curve called A_1. This "fitted" curve is subtracted from the original curve, and the gamma variate is applied to the recirculation component, resulting in a second fitted curve, A_2, that represents recirculation secondary to the shunt (Holman, McNeil, et al., 1976). A_1 is proportional to the pulmonary blood flow while A_2 is proportional to the shunted flow. Thus the Q_p:Q_s flow ratio (pulmonic:systemic flow ratio) was determined as $A_1 \div (A_1 - A_2)$. This method accurately detects and quantitates left-to-right shunts and can separate patients with Q_p:Q_s ratios less than 1:2 from those with ratios over 1:2. Furthermore, it accurately quantitates shunts between 1.2 and less than 3 (Figures 10-4–10-8). The gamma variate method can compute total Q_p:Q_s from areas of interest placed over both lungs or ratios from each lung separately (Figures 10-9 and 10-10). The analysis of the curves assumes that the distribution of flow to the lungs from the right ventricle is not altered during recirculation, but this is not the case in subjects with a patent ductus arteriosus; consequently, different shunt ratios can be determined from each lung in that circumstance (Alazraki, Ashburn, et al., 1972; Maltz and Treves, 1973). Figure 10-10 shows how a similar situation can exist owing to excessive bronchial arterial flow to one lung.

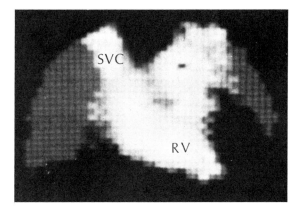

Figure 10-4 The lungs have been outlined by using a light pen for the purpose of creating a time-activity curve of radionuclide passage through the heart. The grey lung zones are the areas of interest in this early image, which shows only lungs and right heart. The lung areas of interest must not overlap other structures such as SVC or RV.

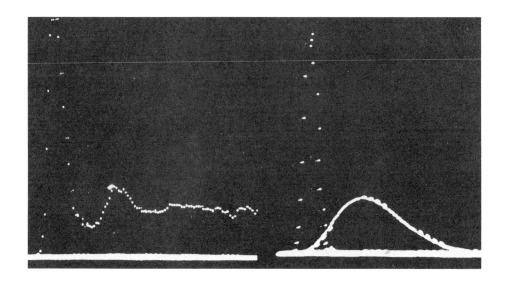

Figure 10-5 Normal pulmonary time-activity curve (each point = 0.5 second). Curve on left is raw curve showing sharp first pass peak, recirculation curve appearing later. Curve on right is processed by gamma variate technique showing two components. The Q_p:Q_s ratio was normal (i.e., 1).

All of these methods, especially the gamma variate technique, are useful in detecting and in some instances quantitating left-ro-right shunts. They are valuable when evaluating children with "innocent" murmurs in whom chest radiograms or electrocardiograms may be normal or equivocal. In such cases, cardiac catheterization may not be warranted and the radio-nuclide shunt study will point to the correct course of action. However, all of these methods have the same limitations as other indicator dilution techniques. Severe aortic or mitral valve insufficiency can cause prolonged pulmonary transit time, which produces a slurred and broadened down-slope in a manner similar to left-to-right shunting. In fact, any condition that prolongs the pulmonary transit time can result in an inconclusive curve analysis. Increased intercostal arterial flow in patients with coarcta-tion of the aorta, significant bidirectional shunting, or a poor, prolonged injection of radionuclide can also render curve analysis difficult if not impossible.

Two other methods have been devised to assist the detection of left-to-right shunting. Goris, Baum, et al. (1976) devised an automatic method of producing parametric images in which tracer progression through the heart is represented by a pseudogrey scale. Areas of interest for curve generation are automatically selected on the basis of peak tracer concen-tration times. Such curves and parametric images have been quite useful in

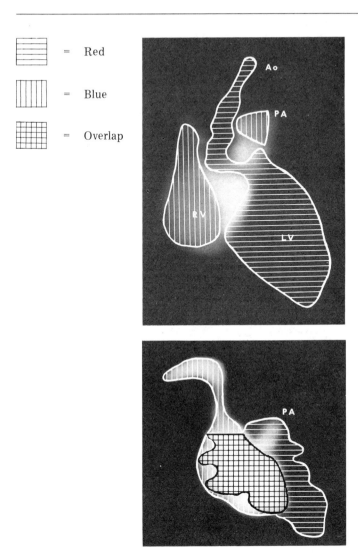

= Red

= Blue

= Overlap

Figure 10-6 Child with cardiac murmur detected by pediatrician during routine physical examination. Chest radiogram and electrocardiogram were normal. In the normal child, nuclear angiocardiogram processed by color-time parametric technique would have shown all cardiac components during the right-heart phase (color-coded blue) as separate from left-sided structures (color-coded red) as shown on top. However, this child (shown on bottom) had filling of the right heart during both phases of the cardiac flow sequence and thus the right and left color codes overlapped, indicating a left-to-right shunt. Notice how the overlapping also extends out into the pulmonary artery and how small the aortic area appears.

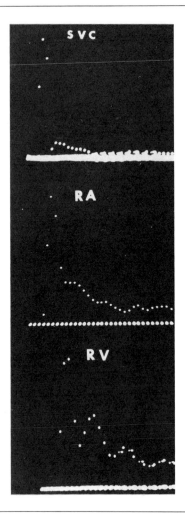

Figure 10-7 In the same patient illustrated in Figure 10-6, areas of interest placed over SVC, RA, and RV showed a sharp spiked curve generated from the SVC region (indicating a good injection), which changed to a slurred curve when the RA and RV regions were studied. This suggested left-to-right shunting at the atrial level (i.e., atrial septal defect, **ASD**).

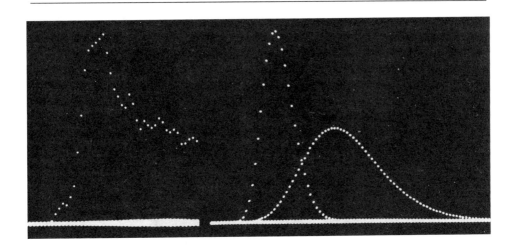

Figure 10-8 In the same patient illustrated in Figures 10-6 and 10-7, pulmonary time-activity curves (raw on left, gamma variate on right) demonstrated abnormal recirculation due to left-to-right shunting. The $Q_p:Q_s$ ratio predicted by this technique was over 2:1. At cardiac catheterization, a 2.3:1 shunt was calculated via the Fick technique. An ASD was also demonstrated.

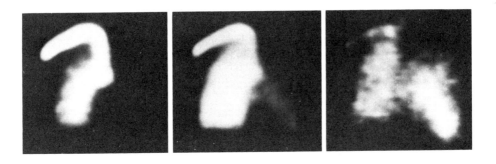

Figure 10-9 Postoperative Glenn procedure (SVC to RPA) for palliation of transposition of the great vessels. Serial images following tracer injection in the right basilic vein showed in sequence: SVC to RL, LV filling, late filling of left lung.

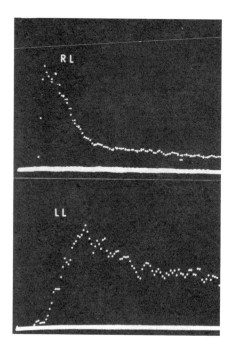

Figure 10-10 In the same patient illustrated in Figure 10-9, time-activity curves were generated from both lungs. Left-to-right shunting was not evident on the right side, but a 3:1 shunt was predicted on the left. The child subsequently underwent surgery for creation of an interatrial baffle, and at operation the surgeon discovered huge bronchial arteries supplying the left lung. This condition, which was similar to a patent ductus arteriosus and explained the predicted shunt, produced a greater left-to-right shunt in the left lung than in the right.

analyzing complex cardiac abnormalities, including those associated with left-to-right shunts. Gates (1978) has used color coding of the right and left heart phases of the cardiac cycle in order to detect overlapping regions that, when present, indicate cardiac chamber filling during both portions of the cycle (Figure 10-6). This technique helps to identify patients with intracardiac left-to-right shunts in circumstances where lung curve analysis may have limitations.

RIGHT-TO-LEFT SHUNT QUANTITATION

Right-to-left shunts can be accurately quantitated following the intravenous injection of 10–15 micron-sized particles of ^{99m}Tc-labeled human albumin microspheres or macroaggregated albumin. Normally 95% of these biodegradable albumin particles impact in the pulmonary arteriolar-capillary bed, producing a "lung scan," while the remaining 5% are diverted into the systemic circulation as a result of intrapulmonary anatomic shunting (Gates and Goris, 1977b). As right-to-left shunting increases, there is a proportionally greater diversion of these radioparticles into the systemic circulation where they transiently impact in the various systemic arteriolar-capillary beds. A total body scintigram should be completed within five minutes of the tracer injection to determine the fraction of the total radionuclide in the body that is located in the systemic circulation. This fraction is proportional to the whole body distribution of net first pass cardiac ejection and is expressed as percent right-to-left shunt as determined by the following formula:

$$\% \text{ R-L shunt} = \frac{\text{Total body count} - \text{Total lung count}}{\text{Total body count}} \times 100$$

A computer or data processing unit is required in order to determine both total body count (obtained either by a moving table or by taking sequential one-minute scintigrams of the entire body) and total lung count. At the same time as the shunt is being calculated, the fractional partition of radionuclide between the lungs is determined (by placing separate areas of interest over each lung) and expressed as the percent interpulmonary distribution of pulmonary arterial (PA) perfusion:

$$\% \text{ PA perfusion to right lung} = \frac{\text{Right lung count}}{\text{Total lung count}} \times 100$$

$$\% \text{ PA perfusion to left lung} = 100\% - \text{Right lung }\%$$

The total albumin injected per test should not exceed 0.2 mg because some of the particles invariably enter the systemic circulation and cause transient arteriolar-capillary blockage. However, these biodegradable particles quickly fragment, pass through the capillary beds, and ultimately are phagocytized by the reticulo-endothelial cells of the liver. This low amount of injectable albumin, which is usually contained in a 0.1 mL volume and injected by tuberculin syringe, gives a safety factor of 6,000-fold (Gates, Orme, et al., 1974). The success of this technique has been validated by comparison with right-to-left shunt calculations obtained at cardiac catheterization by using the Fick technique (Gates, Orme, et al., 1974). The test has been used for nearly 10 years without, to my knowledge, any reported complications.

A few technical or procedural pitfalls deserve mention. If a child is crying or straining at the time of injection and becomes more cyanotic, he or she may increase the calculated shunt in comparison to resting values such as those obtained at cardiac catheterization (Gates, Orme, et al., 1974). Although the calculated value in this situation accurately reflects the physiologic state at the time of injection, it has limited usefulness as

a baseline value for future comparisons. Injection of particles less than
10 μ (which freely pass through the pulmonary capillary bed) or poor
preparations containing unbound ^{99m}Tc will increase the systemic component of the total body count and result in a falsely elevated shunt calculation. Total body scintigraphy should be completed within five minutes
of injection because rapid breakdown of pulmonary particles will result in
progressively increasing systemic counts (Gates and Goris, 1977a). It
matters little whether the total body scan is done anteriorly or posteriorly
as long as it is done promptly. A final word of caution: One should not
inject large particles or ones that break down slowly (e.g., ferric hydrox-
ide) because more proximal, larger-sized vessels will be occluded, or the
transient nature of the temporary blockade will be lost.

The mere detection and quantitation of right-to-left shunting is not
the sole purpose of this study. This technique, which is accurate and easy
to perform, can be done at intervals to permit objective documentation of
the improvement or worsening of cyanotic heart disease—a measure that
is especially useful when following children who have undergone corrective or palliative cardiac surgery. The assessment of the functional state of
a surgically created systemic-pulmonic shunt requires both quantitation of
right-to-left shunting and determination of the interpulmonary distribution of pulmonary perfusion (Figures 10-11 and 10-12). Well-functioning
systemic-pulmonic anastomoses reduce right-to-left shunting by increasing pulmonary flow to each lung, although sometimes unequally. Mal-
functioning anastomoses do not significantly reduce right-to-left shunting and can cause unilateral pulmonary hyperfusion. Nonfunctioning
shunts do not decrease right-to-left shunting but may alter the distribution of pulmonary flow. Perfusion lung scintigrams alone are inadequate
to evaluate shunt function. Preferential radionuclide accumulation can
occur in either lung, regardless of anastomotic function, depending upon
the magnitude of right-to-left shunting, degree of pulmonary outflow obstruction, variability of intercommunication between right and left pulmonary arteries, and the anatomic configuration peculiar to each anastomosis (Gates, Orme, et al., 1975a).

In addition to postsurgical conditions, certain congenital cardiovascular disorders may produce an abnormal perfusion lung scintigram,
usually in the form of maldistribution of pulmonary perfusion (i.e., one
lung receiving at least 30% more perfusion than the opposite side). Such
pulmonary perfusion imbalance may be associated with: branch pulmonary artery stenosis or atresia; patent ductus arteriosus preferentially
perfusing one lung; pulmonary valvular stenosis with selective jetting of
blood to the left lung; or long-standing right ventricular hypertrophy with
twisting of the cardiac axis resulting in selective jetting of blood into the
right lung. Perfusion lung scintigraphy is much more sensitive in detecting
pulmonary flow imbalance than chest radiography. One lung must have at
least two-and-one-half times as much perfusion as the opposite side before
the observer can consistently detect imbalance by inspection of chest

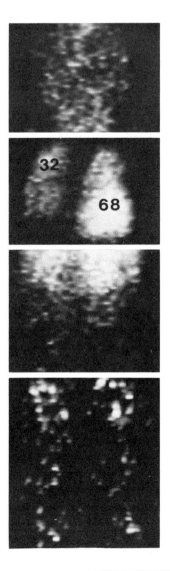

Figure 10-11 Total-body scintigram of a child with tricuspid atresia who had undergone a Waterston anastomosis (Ao to RPA). The scan was posterior. ^{99m}Tc-labeled microspheres had been injected: 33% of the tracer was in the systemic circulation indicating the magnitude of right-to-left shunting. Of total lung radionuclide content, 68% was in the right lung and 32% in the left. This degree of right-to-left shunting and maldistribution of pulmonary perfusion was caused by a twisting of the surgical anastomosis, resulting in its malfunction and the selective hyperperfusion of the right lung by the aorta and the left lung by the pulmonary artery.

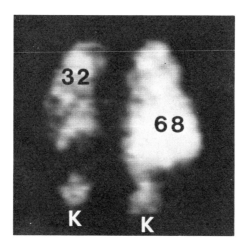

Figure 10-12 Close-up view of lungs showing tracer maldistribution plus kidneys (K) in same patient illustrated in Figure 10-11. Unless there is a right-to-left shunt, renal imaging is never seen on a perfusion lung scintigram performed with a good radiopharmaceutical preparation.

radiograms alone. Likewise, consistent detection of such perfusion maldistribution by cineangiography requires that one lung have at least one-and-one-half times as much perfusion as the opposite side (Gates, Orme, et al., 1975b).

CONCLUSION

The radionuclide assessment of a child with congenital heart disease can be a rewarding experience if the proper tests are performed. The key to success, in addition to the use of modern equipment, is close consultation between cardiologist and nuclear medicine physician. Nuclear medicine personnel must clearly understand the clinical situation if they are to extract the maximum amount of information from each study. These nuclear tests are simple (from the patient's point of view), are accurate, and are easy to perform on an outpatient basis. These features, when combined with their safety, permit their repeated performance, thus allowing for serial follow-up assessments of ill children.

References

Alazraki, N. P.; Ashburn, W. C.; Hogan, A., et al. 1972. Detection of left-to-right cardiac shunts with the scintillation camera pulmonary dilution curves. *J. Nucl. Med.* 13:142–47.

Anderson, P. A. W.; Jones, R. H.; and Sabiston, D. C., Jr. 1974. Quantitation of left-to-right cardiac shunts with radionuclide angiography. *Circulation* 49:512-16.

Gates, G. F. 1978. Assessment of radionuclide angiocardiograms using color/time images. *Radiology* 129:483-87.

Gates, G. F.; and Goris, M. L. 1977a. Suitability of radiopharmaceuticals for determining right-to-left shunting. *J. Nucl. Med.* 18:255-57.

———. 1977b. Hypoxemia unassociated with anatomic shunting. *Clin. Nucl. Med.* 2:227-31.

Gates, G. F.; Orme, H. W.; and Dore, E. K., 1974. Cardiac shunt assessment in children with macroaggregated albumin technetium-99m. *Radiology* 112:649-53.

———. 1975a. Surgery of congenital heart disease assessed by radionuclide scintigraphy. *J. Thorac. Cardiovasc. Surg.* 69:767-75.

———. 1975b. The hyperfused lung: Detection in congenital heart disease. *J.A.M.A.* 233:782-86.

Goris, M. L.; Baum, D.; Wallington, J., et al. 1976. Nuclear angiocardiography: Automated selection of regions of interest for the generation of time-activity curves and parametric image display and interpretation. *Clin. Nucl. Med.* 1:99-107.

Holman, B. L.; McNeil, B. J.; and Adelstein, S. J. 1976. Quantitative tracer kinetics. In *Diagnostic nuclear imaging*, edited by A. Gottschalk and E. J. Potchen, 116-25. Baltimore: Williams & Wilkins.

Jones, R. H.; and Anderson, P. A. W. 1975. Congenital heart disease: Imaging and analytic methods. In *Quantitative nuclear cardiography*, edited by R. N. Pierson, J. P. Kriss, R. H. Jones, et al., 32-65. New York: John Wiley & Sons.

Maltz, D. L.; and Treves, S. 1973. Quantitative radionuclide angiocardiography (determination of $Q_p:Q_s$ in children). *Circulation* 47:1049-56.

Rosenthall, L.; and Mercer, E. N. 1973. Intravenous radionuclide cardiography for detection of cardiovascular shunts. *Radiology* 106:601-06.

11

Uncommon Uses of and Future Trends in Nuclear Cardiology

Victor F. Huckell, M.D.

Assistant Professor of Medicine
University of British Columbia
Vancouver, British Columbia, Canada

This chapter deals with uncommon uses of current nuclear procedures, specifically cardiac masses and tumors, the use of radiolabeled blood cellular components, and positron emission transaxial tomography and myocardial metabolism.

Cardiac masses and tumors involve pericardium, myocardium, and endocardium. The applicability of 99m-technetium pyrophosphate myocardial imaging, gallium-67 imaging, and radionuclide angiography is discussed.

Blood cellular components, specifically white cells and platelets, have been labeled with indium-111. Indium-labeled platelets are being used to evaluate infective endocarditis, intervascular thrombi, and atherosclerosis. This chapter discusses the development of this tool and its future applicability in clinical cardiology.

Positron emission transaxial tomography permits assessment of regional myocardial blood flow, myocardial mechanical function, and regional myocardial metabolism. The potentials of this tool in extending understanding of myocardial metabolism are discussed.

CARDIAC MASSES AND TUMORS

In nuclear medicine, cardiac tumors are most often diagnosed with radionuclide angiocardiography (RNA) and images obtained after the injection of 99m-technetium pyrophosphate (^{99m}Tc-PYP) or thallium-201 (^{201}Tl). However, other less common radiopharmaceuticals have recently gained use in cardiovascular nuclear medicine because of localization in tumors; these include gallium-67 citrate (^{67}Ga), the most widely used tumor (and abscess) seeking radionuclide.

In spite of ^{67}Ga's less-than-optimum physical characteristics (half-life of 78 hours and gamma energies of 93, 184, 296, and 388 kev), suitable images can be obtained with rectilinear scanners or Anger-type scintillation cameras. Doses of 1 to 10 mCi are administered intravenously and the patient is imaged at six to 96 hours after injection. When carrier-free ^{67}Ga is injected, it is protein bound in plasma to transferrin, haptoglobin, and albumin, and is excreted by the renal and colonic routes (Larson, 1978). Its biological distribution, mechanism of localization, and excretion have been extensively reviewed by others (Anghileri and Heidbreder, 1977; Larson, 1978). Although ^{67}Ga is concentrated in tumors, uptake between tumor types, among patients with tumors of the same type, and even between different tumor types in the same patient, can be significantly different (Nelson, Hayes, et al., 1972). Uptake of ^{67}Ga is not specific for neoplasm; increased localization has been observed in a variety of clinical states, including abscess (Littenberg, Taketa, et al., 1973; Gelrud, Arseneau, et al., 1974) and acute myocardial infarction (Kramer, Goldstein, et al., 1974).

In adults, the most common cardiac tumors are metastatic. Primary cardiac tumors appear to be more common than primary pericardial tumors, but a greater proportion of pericardial tumors are malignant (Fine, 1974). Mesothelioma is the most frequently encountered pericardial neoplasm, while the most frequently encountered of all primary cardiac tumors is myxoma in the adults (Fine, 1974). Rhabdomyomas are the most common primary cardiac tumors in infants (Nadas and Ellison, 1968). Although infrequently encountered, sarcomas of muscle origin, either smooth or skeletal, appear to be the most common primary malignant cardiac tumors. In each case, with the use of cardiovascular nuclear medicine techniques, these tumors can be detected by direct uptake of radionuclide, a filling defect on RNA, or as a result of some secondary manifestations such as myocardial necrosis or pericardial effusion.

Pericardium

Involvement of the pericardium by tumor may produce a pericardial effusion with the characteristic "halo" sign on RNA, as previously described (Bonte, 1976; Simpson, 1978). Use of ^{67}Ga in such a patient can reveal diffuse uptake by the pericardium if the effusion contains sufficient inflammatory cells to concentrate the radionuclide adequately. Alternatively, a discrete or localized focus of uptake can represent a metastatic nodule (Simpson, 1978). Positive ^{67}Ga scans, with pericardial involvement by lymphoma (Manfredi, Sundaram, et al., 1978; Yeh and Benua, 1978), malignant melanoma (Yeh and Benua, 1978), and angiosarcoma (Yeh and Benua, 1978), have been reported.

In Hodgkin's disease, cardiac involvement occurs in approximately 10% of cases, the pericardium being the most frequent site. This frequently presents as a "cardiac apical mass" and creates a problem in differentiation from cardiac apical aneurysm, pericardial cyst, and pulmonary atelectasis in the cardiophrenic angle. Gallium-67 imaging is helpful in this differentiation. In addition, ^{67}Ga imaging: (a) helps in staging Hodgkin's disease; (b) is effective in assessing pre- and posttherapy irradiation and chemotherapy; (c) is more reliable in the chest than in the abdomen; and (d) can be used to measure the accuracy of treatment portals, especially in mantle fields encompassing the apical mass and heart (Manfredi, Sundaram, et al., 1978).

Pericardial tumors may be large enough to deform the heart and may involve the wall of the heart and project into cardiac chambers. This produces a filling defect within the cardiac blood pool on RNA, as described for a recurrent pericardial fibrosarcoma (Bonte, 1976). Pericardial lesions resulting from thoracic mass lesions can also be associated with partial or complete obstruction of the superior vena cava (SVC), with demonstration of collateral thoracic veins carrying the radioactive bolus downward past the heart into the subdiaphragmatic region. There may be partial or complete absence of filling of the SVC, late filling of the heart apparently by the inferior vena cava (IVC), and prolongation of total circulation time but with normal right heart-to-aorta circulation time (Kriss, 1969; Matin, Ray, et al., 1970; Kriss, Enright, et al., 1971).

Myocardium

Intramural tumor involving the wall of the left ventricle, and less frequently the right ventricle, can produce a distortion of ventricular anatomy. With first pass RNA, a persistent area of decreased activity can be seen that persists through the dextro (right ventricle) or levo (left ventricle) phase of the cardiac cycle—for example, a myocardial rhabdomyoma (Starshak and Sty, 1978). Another example is right ventricular involvement by metastases from a colonic carcinoma (Steiner, Bull, et al., 1970). Better localization of tumor can be obtained on gated studies with the presence of a persistent filling defect. Involvement of the interventricular septum may be recognized in the left anterior oblique view as a greater-than-normal thickening of the septum with loss of systolic movement.

Replacement of myocardial cells by tumor cells destroys the ability of that portion of the myocardium to localize ^{201}Tl, and the tumor is seen as a "cold spot." In the same situation, ^{67}Ga imaging would demonstrate uptake at the site of the tumor. Diffuse ^{67}Ga uptake is consistent with diffuse pericardial and/or myocardial involvement (Yeh and Benua, 1978), while discrete uptake can represent a pericardial (Simpson, 1978) or myocardial nodule (Manfredi, Sundaram, et al., 1978).

Gallium-67 imaging is a relatively simple and noninvasive procedure, indicated when one suspects cardiac involvement with tumor. It is interesting to speculate that a reasonably well-differentiated rhabdomyoma or rhabdomyosarcoma might have the ability to take up ^{201}Tl (Adelstein and Maseri, 1977) and produce the unusual combination of negative ^{201}Tl images with positive ^{67}Ga images. Finally, sufficient myocardial necrosis can be produced by direct extension of tumor into the heart (Harford, Weinberg, et al., 1977) or by metastases (Soin, Burdine, et al., 1975) to produce false positive ^{99m}Tc-PYP images.

Endocardium

Large filling defects in the cardiac blood pool can be seen on RNA and can be produced by intramural clot (Meek, Brown, et al., 1965), pericardial tumors (Bonte, 1976), myocardial tumors (Yeh and Benua, 1978), right ventricular tumors (Steiner, Bull, et al., 1970), or left ventricular tumors (Isley and Reinhardt, 1962; Bonte and Curry, 1967). Intramural thrombus may also be detected by macroaggregated albumin (MAA), which is trapped by vessel blockage. Freedman (1974) described a patient with trapping of ^{131}I-labeled MAA in the right ventricle during a lung scan after a myocardial infarction. Later, this clump of activity was observed in the lung, after it dislodged from the right ventricle. Thrombus uptake of sulphur colloid can also occur—for example, on indwelling Swan-Ganz catheters, central venous pressure lines, and total parenteral nutrition lines (Figures 11-1 and 11-2).

Some tumors have a rich blood supply and it is occasionally possible to demonstrate this with selective coronary arteriography (Berman, McLaughlin, et al., 1976; Stroobandt, Piessens, et al., 1977). It is also possible to selectively inject with radionuclide-labeled MAA the coronary artery supplying the tumor. Where subsequent images are gated, a relatively immobile hot spot will be seen with sessile tumors, and a mobile hot spot seen with pedunculated myxomas. The hot spot would be seen to move into the region of the ventricle in diastole and into the atrium in systole.

As myxomas are the most common primary cardiac tumors, a more detailed description of the cardiovascular nuclear medicine findings is indicated. These tumors usually occur in the atria and almost invariably

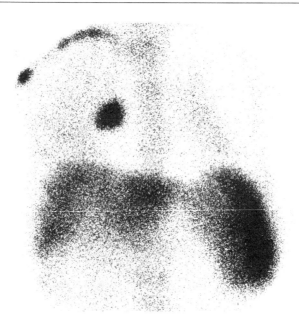

Figure 11-1   Anterior images of a patient with Banti's syndrome. The patient had been on prolonged total parenteral nutrition (TPN). This figure demonstrates intense activity along the TPN line (upper left) and in a thrombus at the tip of the TPN line in the right atrium. The patient subsequently had a small pulmonary embolus, which was documented with ventilation-perfusion imaging.

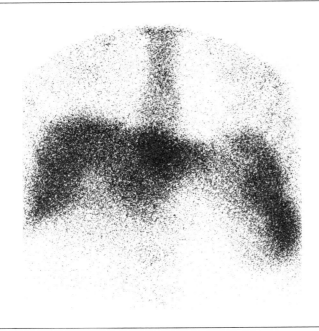

Figure 11-2   Following removal of the TPN line, there is no longer activity in the right atrium.

arise from the interatrial septum; 75% originate from the left atrium. Right atrial myxomas originate from the inferior margin of the fossa ovalis, close to the inferior vena cava, whereas left atrial myxomas arise from the septum primum, at the border of the foramen ovale.

On first pass RNA, a right atrial myxoma shows a space-occupying lesion in the right atrium (Dresser, Rao, et al., 1979) that persists on gated studies. With appropriate views, this filling defect is seen to move to and from the right atrium to the right ventricle (Figures 11-3 and 11-4). Intravenous administration of xenon-133 solution may also demonstrate a large, round filling defect in the region of the right atrium (Meyers, Shapiro, et al., 1977). It is also possible to show prolongation of the time interval necessary to fill the lungs, associated with enlargement of the right atrium, if the right atrial myxoma is sufficiently obstructive in character (Meyers, Shapiro, et al., 1977). Sufficient right atrial outflow obstruction can be produced by a right atrial myxoma to result in enlargement of a patent foramen ovale with right-to-left shunting, detectable on perfusion lung scanning with movement of labeled particles to the left side of the circulation.

Left atrial myxomas were among the first cardiac tumors to be detected by nuclear medicine techniques (Isley and Reinhardt, 1962; Bonte

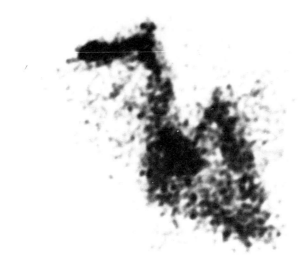

Figure 11-3   First pass radionuclide angiocardiograms performed by injection of 15 mCi of technetium into the right arm. In diastole, there is a well-defined filling defect in the right ventricle below the level of the tricuspid valve.

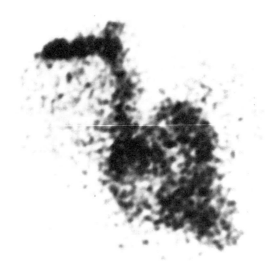

Figure 11-4   In early systole, the filling defect moves up to the low right atrium. Gated radionuclide angiocardiograms also demonstrated movement of the filling defect to and from the right ventricle.

and Curry, 1967). On first pass RNA, a space-occupying lesion of the left atrium may be suspected when there is enlargement of the left atrium, a filling defect in the left atrium, prolonged visualization of the left atrium, and a normal left ventricle (Kriss, Enright, et al., 1971).

Gated RNA permits demonstration not only of the filling defect, but also its characteristic movement to and from the left ventricle (Zaret, Hurley, et al., 1972). Three patterns of movement have been described: (a) a filling defect that moves from the left atrium in end-systole to the left ventricle in end-diastole; (b) a filling defect that remains within the region of the left atrium, but decreases in size between end-diastole and end-systole; and (c) a defect that is observed within the region of the left ventricle in end-diastole but disappears in end-systole (Pohost, Pastore, et al., 1977). Thus, not all myxomas demonstrate movement during the cardiac cycle, and more important, some may appear only in the left ventricle.

Multiple views are necessary to define these filling defects. Gated RNA cardiac blood pool images provide a means of demonstrating myxomas and their position, excursion, and size. The radionuclide approach is less sensitive than echocardiography for myxomas, owing to lower resolution. Myxomas can be missed if composed of multiple small lobules, each of which is too small for resolution by radionuclide techniques. If both echocardiography and RNA are positive, this may be sufficient information to go to surgery without angiographic studies in younger patients (Pohost, Pastore, et al., 1977). Finally, postoperative studies can be of value in demonstrating loss of the filling defect and normal left ventricular function.

In summary, radionuclide techniques dealing with cardiac masses and tumors are still relatively undeveloped. Their use will continue to grow because they are simple, relatively innocuous and noninvasive, and fill a void between clinical examination of the patient and more complicated albeit more definitive procedures such as cardiac catheterization and arteriography. They can be used on an outpatient basis to follow the disease processes over time, in terms of natural history and/or response to therapy.

BLOOD CELLULAR COMPONENTS

The use of radioactively labeled autologous blood cells to define specific pathophysiologic cardiovascular events is based on the work of Thakur, Segal, et al. (1977), who demonstrated that both platelets and polymorphonuclear leukocytes could be labeled with the gamma emitter indium-111 (^{111}In) in a manner that would maintain cellular function as well as allow external imaging with conventional scintillation cameras. Indium-111 is a cyclotron-produced nuclide with a physical half-life of 67.5 hours. It decays by electron capture with two major gamma photons, one at 173 kev (90%) and one at 247 kev (94%) (Thakur, Welch, et al., 1976; Heaton, Davis, et al., 1979).

Initial studies were carried out primarily in animals, but recent studies have extended investigations to humans. Thakur and coworkers compared ^{111}In leukocytes with ^{67}Ga citrate-labeled cells and were able to demonstrate that indium was a better agent for localization of abscesses in dogs. Additional experimental work with ^{111}In-labeled leukocytes has been done in infective endocarditis, myocardial ischemia (in dogs), and experimental myocardial infarction (Thakur, Riba, et al., 1978; Riba, Thakur, et al., 1979a). For example, ^{111}In-labeled leukocyte cardiac imaging did not show any abnormal uptake in rabbits with experimental infective endocarditis. Weiss, Ahmed, et al. (1977) clearly demonstrated accumulation of ^{111}In-labeled white cells in regions corresponding to myocardial infarctions in dogs with experimentally produced coronary occlusion. The positive images correlated well with images obtained with ^{99m}Tc-PYP and computer-reconstructed tomograms obtained with nitrogen-13-labeled ammonia.

Myocardial Infarction

Thakur, Gottschalk, et al. (1979) studied external imaging patterns of kinetics of ^{111}In-labeled polymorphonuclear leukocyte infiltration in the course of the inflammatory response associated with myocardial infarction in dogs subjected to closed chest anterior wall infarction. Maximal epicardial infiltration occurred within the first 24 hours of infarction, while endocardial infiltration was maximal 72 hours after infarction. Leukocyte uptake was minimal in both zones at 120 hours after infarction. In-vivo cardiac images were abnormal, revealing areas of increased myocardial radioactivity in the anterior wall of all dogs studied within 96 hours; all images obtained at 120 hours were negative. In contrast to histopathologic assessments, in-vivo imaging and tissue distribution studies provide direct dynamic data concerning leukocyte infiltration within a given time after infarction. However, Thakur, Gottschalk, et al. felt that their technique would not replace currently available clinical infarct imaging agents (technetium-99m pyrophosphate and thallium-201). Because they were able to relate the kinetics of leukocyte infiltration in infarct zones to both age of the infarct and degree of residual myocardial blood flow, they felt that this tool would be useful for situations of combined old and new infarction where ^{201}Tl imaging might not be diagnostic. In addition, ^{111}In-labeled leukocyte imaging might be of additional value in persistently positive pyrophosphate images caused by either myocytolysis or metastatic calcification (Buja, Poliner, et al., 1977).

Davies, Thakur, et al. (1981) have extended the use of ^{111}In-labeled autologous leukocytes to imaging the inflammatory response in acute myocardial infarction in humans. They have shown that the relationship between image positivity and the temporal imaging sequence is not as distinct as in dogs. In addition, abnormal images were not as discrete in radionuclide uptake. They demonstrated that patients with positive images were injected with labeled cells earlier after infarction than those with negative images. It was felt that this technique could not be applied to the study of patients receiving drug interventions during the early hours of acute infarction. However, the investigators indicated that this technique was useful for the study of the pathophysiology of inflammation in acute infarction.

Infective Endocarditis

Indium-111 platelets have been used to image the lesions of aortic-valve infective endocarditis in a rabbit model (Thakur, Riba, et al., 1978; Riba, Thakur, et al., 1979a). Dramatic images were noted during the first week of the infectious process. This finding was not surprising, since the predominant cellular components of endocardial lesions are bacteria, platelets, and fibrin adherent to damaged valvular endothelium. It was concluded that experimental infective endocarditis could be detected by ^{111}In platelet imaging. However, the lesions produced were relatively large and represented acute fulminant endocarditis. Difference in lesion size between experimental animal and human endocarditis may not allow ready extrapolation to clinical imaging. In addition, in this study it was not clear whether healed or subacute infective endocarditis would concentrate platelets to a comparable degree, or what effect antibiotic therapy would have on platelet deposition. The investigators noted that vegetation uptake was far greater than that reported for venous thrombosis or endarterectomized carotid arteries in dogs (Fuster, Dewanjee, et al., 1978, 1979; Dewanjee, Fuste, et al., 1979).

Intravascular Thrombi

Numerous reports have described the use of radioactive platelets in the detection and localization of experimentally induced and spontaneous vascular lesions in animals and humans (Knight, Primeau, et al., 1977, 1978; McIlmoyle, Davis, et al., 1977a, 1977b; Wistow, Grossman, et al., 1977; Davis, Heaton, Siegel, et al., 1978; Davis, Siegel, Sherman, et al., 1980; Davis, Siegel, and Welch, 1980; Goodwin, Bushberg, et al., 1978; Grossman, Wistow, et al., 1978. Goodwin, Bushberg, et al. (1978) clearly visualized venous and arterial accumulation of radiolabeled platelets in patients with thrombophlebitis, arterial trauma, and recent pulmonary embolism. McIlmoyle, Davis, et al. (1977b) also demonstrated the detection of fresh pulmonary emboli in dogs. They indicated that induced venous thrombi could be scintigraphically detectable by radiolabeled platelet accumulation, with thrombi as old as 72 hours. However, the thrombus-to-blood concentration ratio decreased as a function of thrombus age. They noted that the rapid depletion of extractable thrombin in canine pulmonary emboli suggested that detection of embolism by imaging with ^{111}In-labeled platelets can be limited to relatively new lesions. Anticoagulant therapy can also influence the uptake of labeled platelets by pulmonary emboli. The relationship of thrombus age to uptake of ^{111}In-labeled platelets was also commented on by Knight, Primeau, et al. (1978). In this study, thrombi were removed following provocation and labeling, and then thrombus platelet activity was estimated in an invitro fashion. A 72-hour-old thrombus could not be identified 24 hours after tracer injection (96 hours after thrombus induction), but ^{111}In platelet uptake was still observed in the femoral vein from which the thrombi originated. These findings suggest that imaging will also detect platelet deposition on damaged endothelium in the absence of a fresh thrombus, and have certain implications with regard to the imaging of experimental animals or patients with aortocoronary bypass graft surgery.

However, the debate about whether "old" thrombi can be detected with ^{111}In platelet imaging is a complex one, relating not only to age of the thrombus but also to surface activity. Other studies have clearly demonstrated the detection of left ventricular thrombi 48 months after an acute myocardial infarction. Stratton, Ritchie, et al. (1981) assessed their detection by ^{111}In platelet imaging and compared this method with two-dimensional echocardiography. The latter detected more intracardiac "masses" than platelet imaging, but it was not certain that all of these represented thrombi. This study indicated that, owing to continuing platelet deposition, ^{111}In imaging can detect intracardiac thrombi that have formed remotely in time. It also suggested that optimum imaging time was at least 48 to 72 hours after platelet labeling, and this factor must be considered when reviewing older radiolabeled platelet studies. Ezekowitz, Leonard, et al. (1981) evaluated detection of left ventricular thrombi in patients undergoing aneurysmectomy or valvular replacement. The diagnostic accuracy of platelet scintigraphy in these patients was 100% where surgical or postmortem confirmation of thrombi was obtained. This study permitted the development of preliminary guidelines, making indium platelet scintigraphy a more reliable technique. Many centers use combined indium-111 platelet imaging and 99m-technetium blood pool imaging to permit correction for background activity due to radiolabeled platelets.

Davis and coworkers have evaluated the ability of labeled platelets to detect atherosclerotic lesions in carotid vessels (Davis, Heaton, et al., 1978; Davis, Siegel, et al., 1978; Davis, Siegel, Sherman, et al., 1980; Davis, Siegel, and Welch, 1980). They noted a discrepancy between the degree of "occlusion" as documented by angiography and the intensity of platelet uptake. In addition, they described adherence and aggregation of platelets at atherosclerotic sites as a pathophysiologic process, depending on loss of integrity of arterial endothelial lining. Contrast angiography demonstrates anatomic alterations associated with arterial lesions, but cannot assess thrombotic process dynamics at any given site. Thus, uptake of radiolabeled platelets can reflect "activity" of an arterial lesion rather than the degree of occlusion. The interesting possibility was raised that detection of certain arterial lesions, in spite of concurrent antiplatelet and/or anticoagulant therapy, implies that conventional therapy with such drugs is not optimal, and raises important implications for future investigation and treatment. Also, Davis, Siegel, and Welch (1980) were able to follow the development of an acute arterial thrombus with indium-labeled autologous platelets.

Atherosclerotic Coronary Artery Disease

Riba, Thakur, et al. (1978, 1979a, 1979b) were able to image experimental coronary artery thrombosis in a canine model. Positive platelet images of acute thrombosis, within the left anterior descending coronary artery, could be detected within hours of thrombus formation. Acutely formed thrombi accumulated labeled platelets, but 24-hour-old thrombi did not. Of note was the absence of delayed imaging in these animals. As described earlier, delayed imaging permitted the identification of old left ventricular thrombi and may well permit identification of "older" intracoronary lesions.

A series of studies by Dewanjee and coworkers (Fuster, Dewanjee, et al., 1978, 1979; Dewanjee, Fuster, et al., 1979) has important implications for detection of aortocoronary bypass graft (ACB) occlusion. They studied platelet deposition in patent ACBs in dogs and noted that, even in the presence of patent grafts, the ratio of platelet activity in the graft to blood pool increased with time. Proximal portions of the graft had the highest relative uptake, while the distal portions had relatively lower uptake. Following in-vivo imaging, in-vitro radioactive counting of segments of isolated grafts showed four to 15 times greater activity in the grafts than in blood and 25 to 100 times greater activity than in normal myocardium. The investigators believed that this was sufficient for delineating areas of platelet deposition. A subsequent study replicated the experiment in animals treated with dipyridamole and acetylsalicylic acid (ASA). The animals treated with antiplatelet agents had considerably less platelet deposition as estimated by imaging. This noninvasive technique is therefore a promising tool for studying the role of platelets in the process of saphenous vein bypass graft occlusion in man and its prevention with platelet inhibitors.

A study by Ritchie, Stratton, et al. (1981) assessed the role of dipyridamole plus ASA versus sulfinpyrazone in decreasing platelet deposition in patients with abdominal aneurysms. Sulfinpyrazone appeared to result in decreased platelet deposition in two of four patients, whereas the combination of ASA and dipyridamole had no detectable effect. There is at least one other reported case of a patient with bilateral ulcerated carotid plaques taking ASA and dipyridamole in whom platelet deposition was not prevented (Davis, Heaton, et al., 1978). This unexplained difference between impaired platelet deposition in drug-treated dogs and drug-treated humans may represent a species difference or may simply reflect insensitivity of ^{111}In platelet labeling for detection of minor in-vivo changes. Additional clinical studies are under way.

Thrombi and Prosthetic Materials

A novel use of radiolabeled platelets has been for the in-vivo assessment of the thrombogenicity of cardiovascular catheters (Lipton, Doherty, et al., 1980). Experimental animals were preinjected with radiolabeled auto-logous platelets and a series of catheters were left in situ for 30 minutes to three hours, with sequential external imaging. Lipton and coworkers were able to demonstrate a serial increase in radioactivity over the catheter for up to 40 minutes, with a subsequent plateau. They also demonstrated that catheters with heparin-bonded surfaces had a reduced amount of platelet accumulation. This method has potential use for the clinical study of new catheters and new catheter materials.

The use of radiolabeled platelets will also permit assessment of their deposition on prosthetic grafts such as Dacron. Ritchie, Stratton, et al. (1981) demonstrated platelet deposition on two grafts over one year old, implying a lack of endothelialization in at least some cases. In another study, less ^{111}In platelet activity was found in Gore-Tex femoral arterial implants in dogs treated with dipyridamole (Strathy, Dewanjee, et al., 1980). Thus, platelet imaging holds obvious promise in the in-vivo definition of thrombogenicity of prosthetic graft materials. Finally, because patients with prosthetic grafts retain significant platelet activation, their study can serve as a useful clinical model for the testing of platelet-active drugs (Harker, Slichter, et al., 1977).

POSITRON EMISSION TRANSAXIAL TOMOGRAPHY AND MYOCARDIAL METABOLISM

Positron emission transaxial tomography (PETT) occupies a unique position in nuclear cardiology. This technique permits assessment of regional myocardial blood flow, myocardial mechanical function, and regional myocardial metabolism. A review by Schelbert, Phelps, et al. (1980) dealt with each of these in depth, outlining basic technical aspects, describing quantitative assessment of cardiac performance, and discussing its potential clinical applications.

Physics and Physiology

Positrons are positively charged subatomic particles with mass comparable to that of electrons. When positron-emitting radionuclides give rise to positron particles, the latter lose kinetic energy as they move through matter, owing to interactions similar to those affecting electrons. When the kinetic energy of the positron is almost exhausted, the particle undergoes annihilation by interaction with an electron, resulting in the production of two 511-kev gamma photons emitted in diametrically opposite directions (i.e., at an angle of 180 degrees). Detection of each pair can be accomplished with crystal scintillation detectors oriented 180 degrees apart and connected to a fast coincidence circuit that will record radiation only when both detectors respond simultaneously or within defined limits. The field of view of such a pair of detectors is limited to a cylindrical volume between them providing "electric collimation." In contrast to the field of view of conventional gamma emission detectors, that of electronic collimators is uniform over relatively large distances (Budinger and Rollo, 1977; Phelps, 1977; Weiss, Siegel, et al., 1979).

Variation in counts owing to attenuation—dependent upon the distance of the tracer from the detector—is a significant problem with single photon detectors. With coincident detection, however, the combined attenuation of the two photons, as sensed by both crystals, depends upon the total amount of absorbing material encountered. Thus, when the source is moved closer to one detector, the increased attenuation is offset by a proportional decrease with respect to radiation detected by the other. Accordingly, varying attenuation owing to depth of the tracer within the tissue does not distort the reconstructed image (Ter-Pogossian, Phelps, et al., 1975; Weiss, Ahmed, et al., 1977) as it does with gamma emissions detected with a scintillation camera (Ter-Pogossian, 1976). These properties of positron emission, coupled with the high energy of the photons emitted, facilitate computer reconstruction of positron-emitting radionuclide distribution within a cross-section of the organ of interest. In PETT, each transaxial cross-sectional image is reconstructed from a series of radiation profiles, obtained from pairs of detectors placed around or rotated through selected angles in relation to the organ of interest (Ter-Pogossian, Phelps, et al., 1975).

The major advantages of positron tomography include: (a) development of new positron-emitting radionuclides incorporated into biologically active molecules; (b) the extremely short half-life of most positron-emitting radionuclides, making it possible to use larger amounts to obtain good statistical results at lower total radiation doses and permitting serial studies at short intervals; (c) accurate attenuation correction, allowing the production of images of high quantitative accuracy; and (d) a high detector efficiency, made possible by the elimination of mechanical collimators. This last factor also contributes to superior images, with good statistics at minimal doses of radiation.

However, the same factors that produce certain advantages also result in significant disadvantages. The most useful positron-emitting radionuclides are very short-lived radioisotopes, requiring the ready availability of a cyclotron. Commercially available imaging systems are costly and require unconventional and highly specialized detector systems that are useful only for positron imaging. The extremely short half-life of many of the positron-emitting isotopes also makes them difficult to work with if elaborate mechanical syntheses are required. The high energy of positron-annihilation gamma photons increases the problems of radiation safety and requires special shielding. Finally, the radiopharmaceutical technology required is not commonly available.

Regional Myocardial Blood Flow

Several positron-emitting radiopharmaceuticals have been synthesized for use in assessing myocardial perfusion. Most require an on-site cyclotron because of their short half-lives. Particulate indicators, such as radioactive microspheres, are the most accurate for blood flow measurements. However, their use in human beings is limited because they require administration into the coronary artery, into the left atrium, or at least into the left ventricle (Schelbert, Phelps, et al., 1980). Furthermore, because these indicators are trapped in capillaries, they are of potential risk to organ perfusion (for example, perfusion of the brain).

Rubidium-82, with a half-life of 75 seconds, has been employed in serial studies of regional myocardial perfusion (Beller, Hoop, et al., 1975; Beller, Alton, et al., 1976) using intravenous or intracoronary injection. However, inaccuracies can result because of recirculation and variable extraction of the tracer by ischemic myocardial cells, and because of effects of altered residence time of the tracer (Zaret, 1977). Since extraction increases when residence time is prolonged, diminished uptake by ischemic myocardium can be offset by the increased extraction resulting from prolonged exposure of cell surfaces to the tracer during conditions of low flow.

Another agent used to assess perfusion is 13N-labeled ammonia (13NH$_3$) (Harper, Lathrop, et al., 1972, 1975; Harper, Schwartz, et al., 1973). Its short half-life (10 minutes) permits serial studies. Unfortunately, inhibition of glutamine synthetase leads to a marked reduction in the uptake of 13NH$_3$ by myocardial cells, suggesting that accumulation is dependent upon metabolism as well as perfusion (Harper, Lathrop, et al., 1975). After 13NH$_3$ is incorporated in the large tissue ammonia pool, egress appears to reflect the distribution of myocardial blood flow (Walsh, Harper, et al., 1976). However, apparent perfusion defects may be influenced by relative rates of glutamine synthesis from ammonia. Furthermore, after peripheral intravenous injection, significant incorporation of ammonia in the lungs of heavy smokers may impair delineation of the cardiac uptake and obscure border recognition (Phelps, Hoffman, et al., 1976).

Schelbert, Phelps, et al. (1980) have demonstrated the suitability of this agent to assess regional myocardial flow, both in experimental animals (Gould, Schelbert, et al., 1979) and in human beings (Schelbert, Wisenberg, et al., 1979). They have also shown the potential value of $13NH_3$ and PETT for detecting mild coronary artery stenoses. At rest, coronary blood flow is normal with mild and even moderately severe stenoses. However, coronary flow reserve can be reduced by very mild obstruction, a phenomenon that can be demonstrated during maximal coronary vasodilatation (Gould, Lipscomb, et al., 1974). Schelbert, Phelps, et al. (1980) were able to detect coronary narrowing of less than 50% diameter with $13NH_3$ and PETT during pharmacologically induced vasodilatation (Gould, Schelbert, et al., 1979).

Regional Mechanical Function

Electrocardiographic gated blood pool imaging is now a well-accepted means for determining regional systolic wall motion in the assessment of regional myocardial function (Leitl, Buchanan, et al., 1980). A positron transaxial tomograph can be synchronized with a patient's electrocardiogram and gated cross-sectional images obtained at end-diastole and end-systole, or as a sequence of images throughout the entire cardiac cycle (Weiss, Siegel, et al., 1979). Inhalation of small amounts of carbon-11 carbon monoxide permits very transient labeling of the blood pool by binding to hemoglobin. Using gated cross-sectional images of the cardiac blood pool, quantification of left ventricular wall motion and global left ventricular function is possible (Schelbert, Phelps, et al., 1980).

Wisenberg, Schelbert, et al. (1979) have shown that radioactive counts per minute per gram of tissue increase from end-diastole to end-systole. This increase is proportional to the degree of wall thickening measured echocardiographically. It should therefore be possible to measure regional wall thickening as an index of regional myocardial function. In turn, this will make it possible to correlate this measurement with myocardial blood flow assessed noninvasively.

Regional Myocardial Metabolism

External detection of radioactively labeled free fatty acids (FFA) accumulating in the normal myocardium (Evans, Gunton, et al., 1965) or in normal myocardium surrounding a myocardial infarction (Gunton, Evans, et al., 1965) was among the earliest attempts at myocardial imaging. In 1965, Evans and coworkers showed that radioiodinated long-chain unsaturated fatty acids could be used as imaging tracers for perfused myocardium. Unfortunately, image and data processing equipment available at that time, and the nonavailability of iodine-123, prevented them from following up their initial findings. Of note, metabolic imaging techniques generally employ radioisotopically labeled compounds that are distributed according to regional myocardial perfusion and then become incorporated into various metabolic pathways in the myocardium. The major goal of metabolic imaging is to provide information regarding tissue integrity and viability, as well as information regarding regional perfusion. Major work has been performed in this area using positron-emitting 13NH$_3$ (Walsh, Harper, et al., 1976) and fatty acids labeled with various radionuclides of iodine (gamma emitters) (Evans, Gunton, et al., 1965; Bonte, Graham, et al., 1973; Poe, 1977) or with positron-emitting carbon-11 palmitate (Weiss, Hoffman, et al., 1976; Sobel, Weiss, et al., 1977; Weiss, Ahmed, et al., 1977; Weiss, Siegel, et al., 1977).

Ischemia affects metabolism of FFA in heart muscle by decreasing oxidation and enhancing conversion of substrate to triglycerides (Neely, Rovetto, et al., 1973). In isolated perfused heart studies, Weiss, Hoffman, et al. (1976) demonstrated that consistent depression of FFA extraction was detectable externally in isolated hearts subjected to decreased flow. These observations were subsequently extended to intact dogs with reversible and irreversible coronary occlusion (Weiss, Ahmed, et al., 1977). Zones with decreased positron-labeled FFA accumulation were evident in tomographic images and corresponded to the regions of ischemia supplied by a transiently occluded coronary artery. With irreversible occlusion, there was a persistent defect in accumulation of carbon-11 palmitate. Estimates of infarct sizing, utilizing reconstructed tomograms, correlated closely with morphologic estimates of infarction. These results indicated that necrosis could be quantitatively estimated by noninvasive PETT after the intravenous administration of carbon-11 palmitate to animals with coronary occlusion.

These observations have been extended to patients with acute myocardial infarction at least three months before study (Sobel, Weiss, et al., 1977). Normal subjects exhibited a homogenous distribution of carbon-11 palmitate in tomograms. In patients with transmural myocardial infarction, however, decreased accumulation of palmitate was readily detectable in tomograms.

Single sets of PETT images obtained after intravenous injection of carbon-11 palmitate do not distinguish fresh from old infarction or zones of jeopardized ischemic myocardium from tissue irreversibly injured. However, persistent defects in accumulation are indicative of infarction, and serial tomograms can readily be obtained. Future developments in PETT should permit precise assessment of flow with radiopharmaceuticals presently under development that remain confined to the vascular space.

In summary, fatty acids labeled with short-life positron emitting radionuclides appear to be useful in delineating regional myocardial intermediary metabolism in quantitative terms, and hence in evaluating patients with coronary artery disease and those with other cardiomyopathic processes. Because of its inherent advantages, positron emission tomography will probably become the "gold standard" for noninvasive assessment of myocardial metabolism, under normal and pathologic conditions. However, because of the necessity of having an on-site cyclotron, some centers are evaluating single photon iodine-123 radiolabeled fatty acid imaging for the external assessment of myocardial metabolism in a non-tomographic fashion (Poe, Robinson, et al., 1976; Robinson, 1977; Machulla, Kupsernagle, et al., 1979; Huckell, Lyster, et al., 1979).

References

Adelstein, S. J.; and Maseri, A. 1977. Radioindicators for the study of the heart: Principles and applications. *Prog. Cardiovasc. Dis.* 20:3–17.

Anghileri, L. J.; and Heidbreder, M. 1977. On the mechanism of accumulation of 67 Ga by tumors. *Oncology* 34:74–77.

Beller, G. A.; Alton, W. J.; Moore, R. H., et al. 1976. Detection of nitroglycerin-induced changes in regional myocardial perfusion during acute ischemia by serial imaging with ^{82}Rb^{+}. Abstract, *Circulation* 54 (suppl. II):216.

Beller, G. A.; Hoop, B.; Parker, J. A., et al. 1975. Sequential myocardial imaging with rubidium-82, an ultra-short lived radionuclide. Abstract, *Circulation* 52 (suppl. II):110.

Berman, N. D.; McLaughlin, P. R.; Bigelow, W. G., et al. 1976. Angiographic demonstration of blood supply of right atrial myxoma. *Br. Heart J.* 38:764–66.

Bonte, F. J. 1976. Cardiovascular imaging with radionuclides. In *Diagnostic nuclear medicine*, edited by A. Gottschalk and E. J. Potchen, 149–63. Baltimore: Williams & Wilkins.

Bonte, F. J.; and Curry, T. S. 1967. Technetium-99m HSA blood pool scan in diagnosis of an intracardiac myxoma. *J. Nucl. Med.* 8:35–39.

Bonte, F. J.; Graham, K. D.; and Moore, J. G. 1973. Experimental myocardial imaging with 131 I-labelled oleic acid. *Radiology* 108:195–96.

Budinger, T. F.; and Rollo, F. D. 1977. Physics and instrumentation. *Prog. Cardiovasc. Dis.* 20:19–53.

Buja, L. M.; Poliner, R. L.; Parkey, R. W., et al. 1977. Clinicopathologic study of persistently positive technetium-99m stannous pyrophosphate myocardial scintigrams and mycocytolitic degeneration after myocardial infarction. *Circulation* 56:1016–23.

Davies, R. A.; Thakur, M. L.; Berger, H. J., et al. 1981. Imaging the inflammatory response to acute myocardial infarction in man using indium-111-labeled autologous platelets. *Circulation* 63:826–32.

Davis, H. H.; Heaton, W. A.; Siegel, B. A., et al. 1978. Scintigraphic detection of atherosclerotic lesions and venous thrombi in man by indium-111-labelled autologous platelets. *Lancet* 1:1185–87.

Davis, H. H.; Siegel, B. A.; Heaton, W. A., et al. 1978. Scintigraphic detection of thrombovascular disease utilizing indium-111-labelled autologous platelets. Abstract. In *Proceedings of the second international congress*, World Federation of Nuclear Medicine and Biology, Washington, D.C., 129.

Davis, H. H.; Siegel, B. A.; Sherman, L. A., et al. 1980. Scintigraphic detection of carotid atherosclerosis with indium-labeled autologous platelets. *Circulation* 61:982–88.

Davis, H. H.; Siegel, B. A.; and Welch, M. J. 1980. Scintigraphic detection of an arterial thrombus with In-111-labelled autologous platelets. *J. Nucl. Med.* 21:548–49.

Dewanjee, M. K.; Fuster, V.; Kaye, M. P., et al. 1979. Noninvasive radio-isotopic technique for detection of platelet deposition in coronary artery bypass grafts in dogs and its reduction with platelet-inhibitors. Abstract, *J. Nucl. Med.* 20:604.

Dresser, T. P.; Rao, B. R.; and Winebright, J. W. 1979. Nuclear angiocardiogram to demonstrate right atrial myxoma. *Clin. Nucl. Med.* 4:206–07.

Evans, J. R.; Gunton, R. W.; Baker, R. G., et al. 1965. Use of radioiodinated fatty acids for photoscan of the heart. *Circ. Res.* 16:1–10.

Ezekowitz, M. D.; Leonard, J. C.; Smith, E. O., et al. 1981. Identification of left ventricular thrombi in man using indium-111-labeled autologous platelets: A preliminary report. *Circulation* 63:803–10.

Fine, G. 1974. Primary tumors of the pericardium and heart. In *The heart*, edited by J. E. Edwards and M. Lev, 189–210. Baltimore: Williams & Wilkins.

Freedman, G. S. 1974. Radionuclide angiocardiography in the adult. In *Cardiovascular nuclear medicine*, edited by H. W. Strauss, B. Pitt, and A. E. James, 101–20. St. Louis: C. V. Mosby.

Fuster, V.; Dewanjee, M. K.; Kaye, M. P., et al. 1978. Imaging platelet deposition with 111-In-labeled platelets in coronary artery bypass grafts in dogs. *Mayo Clin. Proc.* 53:327–31.

———. 1979. Noninvasive radioisotopic technique for detection of platelet deposition in coronary artery bypass grafts in dogs and its reduction with platelet inhibitors. *Circulation* 60:1508–12.

Gelrud, L. G.; Arseneau, J. C.; Milder, M. S., et al. 1974. The kinetics of 67-gallium incorporation into inflammatory lesions: Experimental and clinical studies. *J. Lab. Clin. Med.* 83:489–95.

Goodwin, D. A.; Bushberg, J. T.; Doherty, P. W., et al. 1978. Indium-111-labelled autologous platelets for location of vascular thrombi in humans. *J. Nucl. Med.* 19:626–34.

Gould, K. L.; Lipscomb, K.; and Hamilton, G. W. 1974. Physiologic basis for assessing critical coronary stenosis: Instantaneous flow response and regional distribution during coronary hyperemia as measures of coronary flow reserve. *Am. J. Cardiol.* 33:87–94.

Gould, K. L.; Schelbert, H. R.; Phelps, M. E.; et al. 1979. Noninvasive assessment of coronary stenoses by myocardial perfusion imaging during pharmacologic coronary vasodilatation. V. Detection of 47 percent diameter coronary stenosis with intravenous nitrogen-13 ammonia and emission-computed tomography in intact dogs. *Am. J. Cardiol.* 43:200–08.

Grossman, Z. D.; Wistow, E. W.; McAfee, J. G., et al. 1978. Platelets labelled with oxine complexes of Tc-99m and In-111. Part 2. Localization of experimentally induced vascular lesions. *J. Nucl. Med.* 19:488–91.

Gunton, R. W.; Evans, J. R.; Baker, R. G., et al. 1965. Demonstration of myocardial infarction by photoscan of the heart in man. *Am. J. Cardiol.* 16:482–87.

Harford, W.; Weinberg, M. N.; Buja, L. M., et al. 1977. Positive 99m Tc-stannous pyrophosphate myocardial image in a patient with carcinoma of the lung. *Radiology* 112:747–49.

Harker, L. A.; Slichter, S. J.; and Sauvage, L. R. 1977. Platelet consumption by arterial prostheses: The effects of endothelialization and pharmacologic inhibition of platelet function. *Ann. Surg.* 186:594–601.

Harper, P. V.; Lathrop, K. A.; Krizek, H., et al. 1972. Clinical feasibility of myocardial imaging with $^{13}Nh_3$. *J. Nucl. Med.* 13:278–83.

———. 1975. 13N radiopharmaceuticals. In *Radiopharmaceuticals*, edited by G. Subramanian, B. A. Rhodes, and J. F. Cooper, 180–83. New York: Society of Nuclear Medicine.

Harper, P. V.; Schwartz, J.; Beck, R. N., et al. 1973. Clinical myocardial imaging with nitrogen-13 ammonia. *Radiology* 108:613–17.

Heaton, W. A.; Davis, H. H.; Welch, M. J., et al. 1979. Indium-111: A new radionuclide label for studying human platelet kinetics. *Br. J. Haematol.* 42:613–22.

Huckell, V. F.; Lyster, D. M.; and Morrison, R. T. 1979. The potential role of 123 iodine-hexadecenoic acid in assessing normal and abnormal myocardial metabolism. Abstract, *J. Nucl. Med.* 21:57.

Isley, J. K.; and Reinhardt, J. F. 1962. Intracardiac myxoma demonstrated on a vascular scan. *Am. J. Roentgenol.* 88:70–72.

Knight, L. C.; Primeau, J. L.; Siegel, B. A., et al. 1977. Comparison of In-111 labelled platelets and iodinated fibrinogen for the detection of deep vein thrombosis. Abstract, *J. Nucl. Med.* 18:627.

———. 1978. Comparison of In-111-labelled platelets and iodinated fibrinogen for the detection of deep vein thrombosis. *J. Nucl. Med.* 19:891–94.

Kramer, R. J.; Goldstein, R. E.; Hirshfeld, J. W., et al. 1974. Accumulation of gallium-67 in regions of acute myocardial infarction. *Am. J. Cardiol.* 33:861–67.

Kriss, J. P. 1969. Diagnosis of pericardial effusion by radioisotopic angiocardiography. *J. Nucl. Med.* 10:233–41.

Kriss, J. P.; Enright, L. P.; Hayden, W. G., et al. 1971. Radioisotopic angiocardiography: Wide scope in applicability in diagnosis and evaluation of therapy in diseases of the heart and great vessels. *Circulation* 43:792–808.

Larson, S. M. 1978. Mechanisms of localization of gallium-67 in tumors. *Semin. Nucl. Med.* 8:193–203.

Leitl, G. P.; Buchanan, J. W.; and Wagner, H. N. 1980. Monitoring cardiac function with nuclear techniques. *Am. J. Cardiol.* 46:1125–32.

Lipton, M. J.; Doherty, P. W.; Goodwin, D. A., et al. 1980. Evaluation of catheter thrombogenicity in vivo with indium-labelled platelets. *Radiology* 135:191–94.

Littenberg, R. L.; Taketa, R. M.; Alazraki, N. P., et al. 1973. Gallium-67 for localization of septic lesions. *Ann. Intern. Med.* 79:403–06.

Machulla, H. J.; Kupsernagel, C. H.; and Stocklin, G. 1979. Comparative studies of 123 I-fatty acids in myocardial metabolism: Development of omega-123 I-heptadecenoic acid and clinical application for in-vivo diagnosis. *J. Lab. Comp. Radiopharmacol.* 16:75–76.

McIlmoyle, G.; Davis, H. H.; Welch, M. J., et al. 1977a. Diagnosis of experimental pulmonary emboli with indium-111 labelled platelets. Abstract, *J. Nucl. Med.* 18:627.

———. 1977b. Scintigraphic diagnosis of experimental pulmonary embolism with In-111-labelled platelets. *J. Nucl. Med.* 18:910–14.

Manfredi, I. L.; Sundaram, R.; Ramadan, F. M., et al. 1978. 67 Ga scintigraphy in lymphomas with special reference to cardiac apical mass. *Clin. Nucl. Med.* 3:43–47.

Matin, P.; Ray, G.; and Kriss, J. P. 1970. Combined superior vena cava obstruction and pericardial effusion demonstrated by radioisotopic angiocardiography. *J. Nucl. Med.* 11:78–80.

Meek, D. C.; Brown, D. W.; Shmock, C. L., et al. 1965. Demonstration of ventricular aneurysms by radioisotope scanning. *Radiology* 5:856–59.

Meyers, S. N.; Shapiro, J. E.; Barresi, V., et al. 1977. Right atrial myxoma with right to left shunting and mitral valve prolapse. *Am. J. Med.* 62:308–14.

Nadas, A. S.; and Ellison, R. C. 1968. Cardiac tumors in infancy. *Am. J. Cardiol.* 21:363–66.

Neely, J. R.; Rovetto, M. J.; Whitmer, J. T., et al. 1973. Effects of ischemia on function and metabolism of the isolated working rat heart. *Am. J. Physiol.* 225:651–59.

Nelson, B.; Hayes, R. L.; Edwards, C. L., et al. 1972. Distribution of gallium in human tissues after intravenous adminstration. *J. Nucl. Med.* 13:92–100.

Phelps, M. E., 1977. Emission computed tomography. *Semin. Nucl. Med.* 7:337–65.

Phelps, M. E.; Hoffman, E. J.; Coleman, R. E., et al. 1976. Tomographic images of blood pool and perfusion in brain and heart. *J. Nucl. Med.* 17:603–12.

Poe, N. D. 1977. Rationale and radiopharmaceuticals for myocardial imaging. *Semin. Nucl. Med.* 7:7–14.

Poe, N. D.; Robinson, G. D.; Graham, L. S., et al. 1976. Experimental basis for myocardial imaging with 123-I-labelled hexadecenoic acid. *J. Nucl. Med.* 17:1077–82.

Pohost, G. M.; Pastore, J. O.; McKusick, K. A., et al. 1977. Detection of left atrial myxoma by gated radionuclide cardiac imaging. *Circulation* 55:88–92.

Riba, A. L.; Thakur, M. L.; Gottschalk, A., et al. 1978. Imaging of acute coronary artery thrombosis with indium-111 platelets. Abstract, *Circulation* 58 (suppl. II):4.

———. 1979a. Imaging experimental infective endocarditis with indium-111-labeled blood cellular components. *Circulation* 59:336–43.

———. 1979b. Imaging experimental coronary artery thrombosis with indium-111 platelets. *Circulation* 60:767–75.

Ritchie, J. L.; Stratton, J. R.; Thiele, B., et al. 1981. Indium-111 platelet imaging for detection of platelet deposition in abdominal aneurysms and prosthetic arterial grafts. *Am. J. Cardiol.* 47:882–89.

Robinson, G. D. 1977. Synthesis of 123 I-16-iodo-9-hexadecenoic acid and derivatives for use as myocardial perfusion imaging agents. *Int. J. Appl. Radiat. Isot.* 28:149–56.

Schelbert, H. R.; Phelps, M. E.; Hoffman, E., et al. 1980. Regional myocardial blood flow, metabolism and function assessed noninvasively with positron emission tomography. *Am. J. Cardiol.* 46:1269–77.

Schelbert, H. R.; Wisenberg, G.; Gould, L., et al. 1979. Detection of coronary artery stenosis in man by positron emission computed tomography and N-13 ammonia. Abstract, *Circulation* 60 (suppl. II):60.

Simpson, A. J. 1978. Malignant pericardial effusion diagnosed by combined 67 Ga-citrate and 99m Tc-pertechnetate scintigraphy. *Clin. Nucl. Med.* 3:445–46.

Sobel, B. E.; Weiss, E. S.; Welch, M. J., et al. 1977. Detection of remote myocardial infarction in patients with positron emission transaxial tomography and intravenous 11-C palmitate. *Circulation* 55:853–57.

Soin, J. S.; Burdine, J. A.; and Beal, W. 1975. Myocardial localization of 99m Tc-pyrophosphate without evidence of acute myocardial infarction. *J. Nucl. Med.* 16:944–46.

Starshak, R. J.; and Sty, J. R. 1978. Radionuclide angiography: Use in the detection of myocardial rhabdomyoma. *Clin. Nucl. Med.* 3:106–07.

Steiner, R. M.; Bull, M. I.; Kumpel, F., et al. 1970. The diagnosis of intracardiac metastasis of colon carcinoma by radioisotopic and roentgenographic studies. *Am. J. Cardiol.* 26:300–04.

Strathy, K. M.; Dewanjee, M. K.; Kaye, M. P., et al. 1980. Quantitation of platelet deposition in Gore-Tex femoral artery implants in the canine model and its reduction with dipyridamole and prostacyclin. Abstract, *Am. J. Cardiol.* 45:424.

Stratton, J. R.; Ritchie, J. L.; Hamilton, G. W., et al. 1981. Left ventricular thrombi: In vivo detection by indium-111 platelet imaging and two dimensional echocardiography. *Am. J. Cardiol.* 47:874–81.

Stroobandt, R.; Piessens, J.; and DeGeest, H. 1977. Arterial blood supply to a left atrial myxoma diagnosed by coronary arteriography: Report of a case. *Eur. J. Cardiol.* 5/6:477–80.

Ter-Pogossian, M. M. 1976. Limitations of present radionuclide methods in the evaluation of myocardial ischemia and infarction. *Circulation* 53 (suppl. I):119–21.

Ter-Pogossian, M. M.; Phelps, M. E.; Hoffman, E. J., et al. 1975. A positron-emission transaxial tomograph for nuclear imaging (PETT). *Radiology* 114:89–98.

Thakur, M. L.; Gottschalk, A.; and Zaret, B. L. 1979. Imaging experimental myocardial infarction with indium-111-labeled autologous leukocytes: Effects of infarct age and residual regional myocardial blood flow. *Circulation* 60:297–305.

Thakur, M. L.; Riba, A.; Bushberg, J., et al. 1978. Cardiac imaging with indium-111 labelled blood components. Abstract. In *Proceedings of the second international congress*, World Federation of Nuclear Medicine and Biology, Washington, D.C., 129.

Thakur, M. L.; Segal, A. W.; Louis, L., et al. 1977. Indium-111 labeled cellular blood components: Mechanism of labelling and intracellular location in human neutrophils. *J. Nucl. Med.* 18:1020–24.

Thakur, M. L.; Welch, M. J.; Joist, J. H., et al. 1976. Indium-111 labelled platelets: Studies on preparation and evaluation of in vitro and in vivo functions. *Thromb. Res.* 9:345–57.

Walsh, W. F.; Harper, P. V.; Resnekov, L., et al. 1976. Noninvasive evaluation of regional myocardial perfusion in 112 patients using a mobile scintillation camera and intravenous nitrogen-13 labeled ammonia. *Circulation* 54:266-75.

Weiss, E. S.; Ahmed, S. A.; Thakur, M. L., et al. 1977. Imaging of the inflammatory response in ischemic canine myocardium with 111-indium-labeled leukocytes. *Am. J. Cardiol.* 40:195-99.

Weiss, E. S.; Ahmed, S. A.; Welch, M. J., et al. 1977. Quantification of infarction in cross sections of canine myocardium in vivo with positron emission transaxial tomography and 11-C palmitate. *Circulation* 55:66-73.

Weiss, E. S.; Hoffman, E. J.; Phelps, M. E., et al. 1976. External detection and visualization of myocardial ischemia with ^{11}C-substrates in vitro and in vivo. *Circ. Res.* 39:24-32.

Weiss, E. S.; Siegel, B. A.; Sobel, B. E., et al. 1977. Evaluation of myocardial metabolism and perfusion with positron-emitting radionuclides. *Prog. Cardiovasc. Dis.* 20:191-206.

———. 1979. Evaluation of myocardial metabolism and perfusion with positron-emitting radionuclides. In *Principles of cardiovascular nuclear medicine*, edited by B. L. Holman, E. H. Sonnenblick, and M. Lesch, 66-82. New York: Grune & Stratton.

Wisenberg, G.; Schelbert, H.; Selin, C., et al. 1979. The use of positron emission tomography to quantify regional myocardial blood flow. Abstract, *Circulation* 60 (suppl. II):268.

Wistow, B. W.; Grossman, Z. D.; Subramanian, G., et al. 1977. Technetium-99m-oxine and indium-111-oxine labelled autologous platelets: Demonstration of fresh experimental venous thrombi in the rabbit and dog. Abstract, *J. Nucl. Med.* 18:627-28.

Yeh, S. D. J.; and Benua, R. S. 1978. Gallium-67-citrate accumulation in the heart with tumor involvement. *Clin. Nucl. Med.* 3:103-05.

Zaret, B. L. 1977. Myocardial imaging with radioactive potassium and its analogs. *Prog. Cardiovasc. Dis.* 20:81-94.

Zaret, B. L.; Hurley, P. J.; and Pitt, B. 1972. Non-invasive scintiphotographic diagnosis of left atrial myxoma. *J. Nucl. Med.* 13:81-84.

Index